SECRETS OF
ABORIGINAL HEALING

"In this dramatic and inspiring book Gary Holz charts a course on how intuition, surrender, and willingness are essential to the heroic journey of healing oneself."

WARD SERRILL, FILMMAKER, DIRECTOR, AND WRITER OF THE AWARD-WINNING FILM *THE HEART OF THE GAME*

". . . allows us a special glimpse into the heart of the Aboriginal world. It offers us insights into an ancient system of healing that touches on all aspects of wellness, from the physical to the spiritual to the emotional."

JOY PARKER, COAUTHOR OF *WOMAN WHO GLOWS IN THE DARK* AND *MAYA COSMOS*

"This story inspires us to engage our own life more fully—to awaken our own inner capacity for well-being—no matter where we find ourselves."

JIM MACARTNEY, AUTHOR OF *CRISIS TO CREATION: OUR POWER OF CHOICE*

"Anyone who needs to heal would enjoy this book."

KRYSTA GIBSON, EDITOR OF *NEW SPIRIT JOURNAL*

"What so many of us seek is not more information but guided wisdom that resonates with a deep place in our soul. One of love, nurturing, and truth that acts as another breadcrumb on the path to our true selves and healing at all levels. Robbie and Gary Holz's footsteps on this sacred journey are what they share with readers in this book and in their work."

RIK ROBERTS, PSYCHOLOGIST AND RETIRED JOURNALIST

"Different from most self-help books, *Secrets of Aboriginal Healing* gives a more personal voice to learning about the healing powers we each have inside of us."

PAT RATLIFF, EDITOR OF *EDMONDS BEACON*

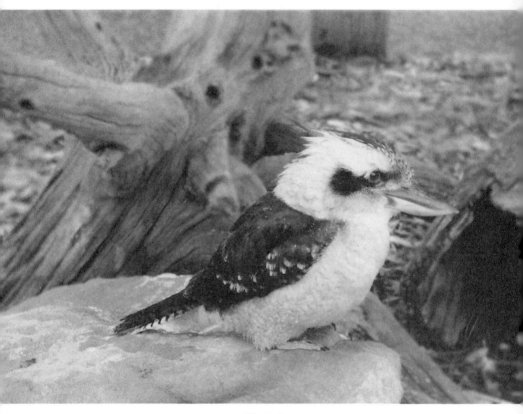
Kookaburra.
Photograph by Robbie Holz.

SECRETS OF
ABORIGINAL HEALING

A PHYSICIST'S JOURNEY WITH A REMOTE AUSTRALIAN TRIBE

GARY HOLZ, D.Sc.,
WITH ROBBIE HOLZ

Bear & Company
Rochester, Vermont • Toronto, Canada

Bear & Company
One Park Street
Rochester, Vermont 05767
www.BearandCompanyBooks.com

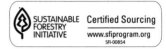

Text stock is SFI certified

Bear & Company is a division of Inner Traditions International

Library of Congress Cataloging-in-Publication Data
Holz, Gary, 1950–2007.
  Secrets of aboriginal healing : a physicist's journey with a remote Australian tribe / Gary Holz, D.Sc., with Robbie Holz.
    pages cm
  Summary: "A guide to the 60,000-year-old healing system of the Aborigines revealed through one man's journey to overcome multiple sclerosis"— Provided by publisher.
  ISBN 978-1-59143-175-6 — ISBN 978-1-59143-753-6 (e-book)
  1. Aboriginal Australians—Health and hygiene. 2. Aboriginal Australians—Medicine—History. 3. Spiritual healing—Australia. 4. Multiple sclerosis—Alternative treatment. I. Holz, Robbie, 1954- II. Title.
  RA553.H65 2013
  362.1968'340092—dc23
  [B]
                                                                2013009997

Printed and bound in the United States by Lake Book Manufacturing, Inc. The text stock is SFI certified. The Sustainable Forestry Initiative® program promotes sustainable forest management.

10 9 8 7 6 5

Text design and layout by Brian Boynton
This book was typeset in Garamond Premier with Gill Sans as a display typeface

To send correspondence to the author of this book, mail a first-class letter to the author c/o Inner Traditions • Bear & Company, One Park Street, Rochester, VT 05767, and we will forward the communication, or contact the author directly at **www.holzwellness.com.**

To Chris and Sonia, the driving force in the quest to become whole again, and who remain a larger part of our hearts than they can ever imagine;

To Robert and Marge, who exemplify extraordinary love and service to community;

To Corey, a constant source of inspiration and loved more than words can possibly express;

To Laurie, a shining heart and one of the greatest blessings in our lives;

To Rose and Ray, who were the guides on an incredible journey;

To the remote Outback Aborigines, who so generously shared their healing knowledge;

To all those who suffer but refuse to give up hope, even though others have told them their case is hopeless;

And to the Big Guy—who is in charge of it all.

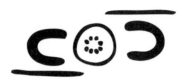

This book exists because of many wonderful people in our lives. Their skills, love, and support helped in one form or another in the birthing of this book.

We acknowledge and hold much gratitude in our hearts for them, especially the following: Ron and Barbara Carstens, Kathy Logan, Ouida Shelton, Dee Griffin, Joy Parker, Sara Stamey, Theresa Black-McCartney, Mary, Danielle Gibbons, Raven Neumann, Kim Votry, Starfeather, Christiann Howard, Adrienne Fermoyle, and our family and friends.

CONTENTS

FOREWORD

BY JOY PARKER

When I first met Gary Holz in 1995, I was immediately fascinated with his extraordinary story about the time he spent with the Aborigines in the Australian Outback. One of the questions a reader might ask upon reading that account in this book is: "Is this a true story? Are the people and events that Gary describes real? How is it that the two Aboriginal medicine people spoke English and used modern words such as 'programming' and 'the subconscious'?"

Since 1983 I have worked as an editor and cowriter with anthropologists, indigenous healers, and medicine people. I learned how these sorts of people live and travel between the traditional village and the modern Westernized city. When I read about Ray and Rose, the two Aboriginal healers who worked with Gary in the Outback, I immediately recognized them as being typical of the indigenous person who is adept at moving between the "two worlds." Many of these people have assumed this role because the time has come for them to share with the outside world their knowledge, which their people have kept hidden for centuries.

Westerners often have misconceptions about the indigenous. We are frequently conditioned to believe that people born in remote villages, like those in the Australian Outback, are "primitives" who know very little about Western culture. Mayan shaman Martín Prechtel often jokes that people expect him to "talk like Tarzan" and to be naive about things like history and politics. Among other accomplishments, Martín is an expert in sixteenth-century history and speaks several languages.

There are thousands of indigenous people who work in the modern city but still regard the village as home. Some of them, like Gary's Aboriginal healer Rose, were born in the city (Brisbane) of an indigenous parent and a white parent and therefore speak a Western language fluently. Yet they prefer spending most of their time in the village of their tribe of origin.

We know that, in spite of all the benefits of "civilization," there is something that we are still lacking. We want to hear again the voices of our own ancestors—the songs they sang when they lived in harmony with the Earth—in the village of our own ancient memory. That's why we read books like *Secrets of Aboriginal Healing;* that's why we love stories like the one that Gary tells here.

Over the past several years many indigenous cultures have come forward and told their stories and shared their medicine. *Secrets of Aboriginal Healing* is another strand of this great tapestry, what the Mayans called "the story of the original flowering Earth." This book allows us a special glimpse into the heart of the Aboriginal world. Most important, it offers us insights into an ancient system of healing that touches on all aspects of wellness, from the physical to the spiritual to the emotional.

Secrets of Aboriginal Healing is a great gift. By sharing his own story with such openhearted honesty, Gary has given us a mirror in which to see our own wounded souls and a map to find our way back home. We are fortunate indeed to receive his words.

JOY PARKER is a writer, editor, and popular lecturer. She is the coauthor of two groundbreaking books on the history of the Maya Indians, *A Forest of*

Kings and Maya Cosmos. More recently, she coauthored *Woman Who Glows in the Dark.*

Ms. Parker has made television appearances related to her expertise in indigenous tribes. She has taught at both New York University and Columbia University and currently teaches at the University of California at Irvine.

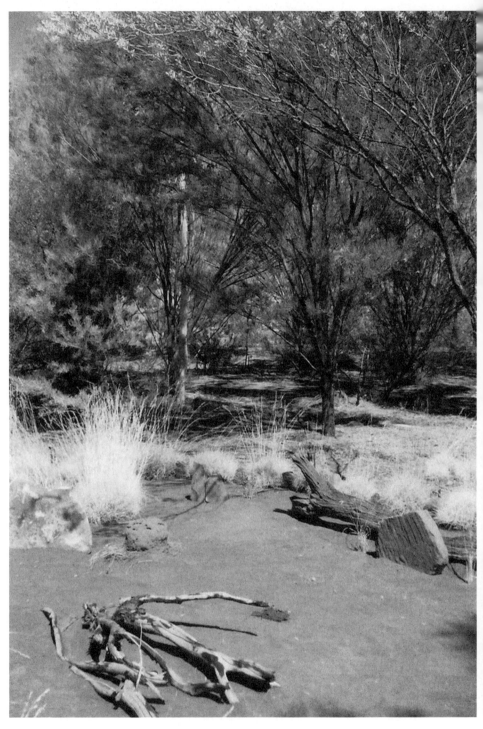

Outback desert, similar to the setting of Gary Holz's Aboriginal experience.
Photo by Robbie Holz.

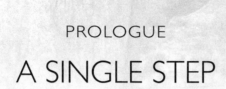

A SINGLE STEP

According to my doctors, I was not supposed to be alive today. But I am. Why I am and how I got well, how I was healed, has been for me a revelation. And a miraculous journey. What I've learned about healing you can learn, too, if you're willing.

The healing I experienced was not done through modern medicine, with wonder drugs and technologies. No. For me the healing began on the other side of the world, in the Australian Outback. With ways that are as ancient as the human race itself.

The trip to the Outback began with a single step—a step I took on my way to yet another business meeting. A step when my left foot didn't lift properly. I noticed that I was dragging it a little as I walked. For most people this would have been a clear warning that something was wrong. But my life had enough problems. I must have strained a muscle, I told myself. The next day my foot was normal, and I forgot about it.

But then the "dragging" returned. More insistently. The scuff marks across the top of my shoes proved I wasn't imagining the weakness in the left foot. And the tingling numbness wasn't imagination either. It was real. Too real. I thought about it and decided I had pinched a nerve in my foot and it would disappear in time.

For several months I experienced a period of numbness and tingling in my left leg, followed by a period of normalcy. I could live with the temporary discomfort, but was troubled that the area of numbness was increasing. It worked its way from the left foot to the left calf, then started in the right foot and worked its way to the right calf.

At the time my high-tech aerospace company was growing rapidly and demanding most of my time and attention. My troubled marriage gave me even more motivation to stay focused on my business and stay on the road. I had no time for symptoms, for pinched nerves, for any distraction. So I bought a cane at a local drug store.

I would have continued living this way indefinitely if I hadn't awakened one morning and discovered that the numb feeling now had me by the short hairs. It had spread to my groin area. It was taking over my sense of maleness. A cane was one thing, but this was something altogether different. I called that day and arranged to take tests at Scripps Clinic in La Jolla, near San Diego.

What happened next knocked the wind out of me. The doctor advised, "At this point the most educated guess says you are suffering from chronic progressive MS—multiple sclerosis." He cautioned that it was not easy to diagnose my symptoms, but the huge battery of tests that I had taken strongly pointed to MS.

I was speechless. All I could do was cling to the words "educated guess." Maybe he was wrong. My mind began scrambling for loopholes. This doctor had admitted that multiple sclerosis was difficult to diagnose. I could be suffering from stress—perhaps from the turbulence in my family life. My first marriage had ended in divorce and my second marriage was rapidly heading for the same rocks. My children from the first marriage were cold and distant. And there was the constant pressure of running my business. Surely that was enough to cause some stress-related symptoms. That was it, I was certain. I just needed some rest, an escape from the stress for a while. Then I'd feel healthy again.

As my mind continued to marshal its arguments, the doctor continued. "We can give you medication that will ease the pain. Unfortunately, there is no known cause for multiple sclerosis, and therefore we have no cure."

No cure.

Those two words stopped the chatter of my mind and began to repeat like a broken record. *No cure. No cure.* The doctor droned on in a voice so flat he could have been lecturing to a classroom of bored medical students.

"Many of the characteristics of this disease suggest that it is an auto-immune disorder. In other words, antibodies begin to attack the cells that make myelin in the fluid surrounding your brain and the nerves of the spinal cord. When that myelin is destroyed, your body replaces it with a scarlike material we call plaque. As this layer of plaque accumulates, the function of that particular nerve system deteriorates."

He recited that there would be periods when I would experience an increase in pain and a worsening of symptoms—an "exacerbation." Although it was a temporary state and the symptoms would decline in intensity with time, there would sometimes be a permanent result such as numbness.

Then in a slightly softer voice—as if he finally remembered he was talking to the patient, the one for whom there was "no cure," rather than a class of students—he added, "I know it's no comfort but the reality is, we simply don't know yet how this will affect your life. The course of the disease varies from person to person. It is impossible to know what course yours will take or how severe it will become."

Even though I needed to hear what he said, it was too difficult to listen. I seemed to be outside myself, watching the entire scene from someplace else—someplace safe. In the strangest way I was fully aware yet absent. Where was my reaction to this news? I should have been horrified. But somehow, no emotions came. I felt no fear, no anger, no self-pity, no sorrow. I felt nothing. Just emptiness.

The next seven years of my life were a nightmare. The symptoms worsened. I began taking Prednisone, a powerful steroid that had debilitating side effects. All the doctors could do for me was to increase the dosage of my medication, which had less and less effect as time went on. Eventually, I was being hospitalized every six or seven months.

For four years I continued dragging myself around airports and boardrooms, forcing myself to "walk" on two canes because I was afraid that once I got into a wheelchair I'd never get out again. Finally, in 1988, I gave in. I got a chair. That was also the year that I began taking a liter of Prednisone a day through an IV. I thought things couldn't get much worse.

But they did. In 1994 my doctor told me that I was losing the battle. My internal organs were shutting down. I should begin to get my affairs in order. He cautioned that I had two years to live—at most.

Two years. I was 43 years old and had two years to live. I received my death sentence with despair. By then I was spending most of my time in a wheelchair, had almost no feeling in my body, was catheterized, and could barely lift my arms to feed myself. Even so, I knew I was not ready to die. There was still so much that I wanted to experience.

And so I grieved. I grieved for the loss of things large and small. Like wading in the ocean and feeling the gentle touch of the water on my toes. Like bouncing a grandchild upon my knee. Like making love. My desperation was deep and black, and I felt totally alone.

And then there occurred a series of what I would have called strange coincidences, except that I have since come to believe that there are no coincidences. Seeking relief from the unrelenting depression, I stopped in at a local jazz club. Perhaps the music would take my mind off my problems. It was so crowded that I almost turned back, but somehow I felt compelled to go in.

Precisely because it was so crowded, I ended up talking to a woman from Australia. She happened to be a naturopath. We happened to talk about alternative healing methods, and especially those of the Australian Aboriginal people. She happened to know some extraordinary healers in an Aboriginal tribe in the Australian Outback. She happened to have the phone number of one, Ray Gelar, who spent part of his time in Brisbane. She happened to give it to me.

That was strange enough, but even stranger is that I had a strong urge to call him. It was completely out of character for me, but I did it. I called Ray. I asked him if he could help me. And although, as I found later, he and other healers in his tribe did not normally work with outsiders, he agreed to work with me.

A week later, this man who had devoted his life to physics, to logic, to hard cold facts, rolled his wheelchair onto a plane bound for Australia. My family thought I was insane. There was a part of me that thought

I was insane. But another part of me was saying that this was my only chance. What did I have to lose?

At the end of a grueling flight, sitting upright in my wheelchair for more than 18 hours, I was met in Brisbane by Ray. He told me that he was taking me to a village in the Outback where I would be working directly with another healer, a woman named Rose, and that he would assist her. A seven-hour drive brought us to the village, where I met Rose and began the work of healing. She told me that the Aboriginal people do not run a clinic out of their village. They do not treat outsiders, but they had agreed to treat me. In fact, she told me that I was the first outsider in over forty years with whom this tribe had shared their medicine.

When I asked Rose why I had been allowed to come, she stated simply that the "Big Guy"—God—had told them that someone was coming from the West and that they should get ready for him.

Under Rose's care I began working eight to ten hours a day with the 50,000-year-old Aboriginal system of emotional, spiritual, and physical healing. Within a short time I experienced the first miracle—sensation began to return to my body! The following days were joyful. I first began by moving parts of my body that had been paralyzed for many years. Then I became able to stand and, with some support, to walk.

As my body continued to heal, I was summoned to a meeting with Old Healer, the ancient Aboriginal elder who supervised my treatment with Rose. Old Healer told me that not only was I going to recover from my illness but that I was destined to help others. "Someday you will be a powerful healer," he proclaimed. "You have enough power in your body to light up a small city." For the rest of my stay, he revealed, I would be learning not only how to heal myself, but also how to heal others.

During my time in the Outback, I not only regained my health, but also found my life's work as a healer and a teacher of this ancient medicine. Before I left Australia I made a commitment to my Aboriginal friends that I would share with others the gift of healing techniques they had shown me. I also promised to explore and develop my own healing gift.

After my return to the United States in 1994, I continued to recover and strengthen my body while I earned a Master's degree in Nutrition and a Doctorate of Science in Immunology. I wanted to see how Western medicine could complement the ancient healing secrets of the Aboriginal people. I then opened a clinic and began working with those who needed healing. Since then I have relieved the symptoms of terminal diseases such as cancer and HIV/AIDS, as well as chronic illnesses like macular degeneration, arthritis, and scoliosis.

Aboriginal medicine offers us much that is unique. I was a man who had devoted his life to intellectual pursuits, following the logic of the head. What I found in the Outback was a system that could teach me to know and trust the wisdom of the heart. It was a system that was strong enough and thorough enough to transform my entire way of looking at life, for it was really my belief system that was manifesting as MS in my body and literally killing me.

Although the actual names of the people written about in this book have been changed to protect their privacy, the materials from my discussions with the Aboriginal people are quoted exactly since I took a voice-activated tape recorder to the Outback to preserve my experiences. I originally created the recordings for my children, so that after my death, they might better understand me. I did not want to leave this life without making one final effort to bridge the gap between us. Little did I know that I not only would live to be reunited with my children, but that the recordings would be used for a higher purpose—to help heal others as I had been healed.

I know that the healing secrets of the Aboriginal people have worked not only for me but also for thousands of others. I want to share them with as many people as I can. The most important thing I want to communicate through telling my story is that there's hope for you—no matter what illness you might have—if you are willing to search for answers. If modern medical science has done all it can for you and you are still not well, seek out alternatives. In 1994 I was given two years to live. Many years later I'm still here. I am living proof that there is always hope if we can just journey to the heart.

I

THE OUTBACK

After more than 18 hours of plane travel, all of it sitting upright in my wheelchair, I was finally in the Brisbane airport. A steward had collected my luggage and pushed me to a payphone so that I could call Ray, my only contact on this immense continent. I had been unable to get any sleep for the entire trip, and now the combination of exhaustion and apprehension began to catch up with me. Everything felt surreal as I dialed the number.

Just over a week earlier I had been sitting in a jazz lounge, talking to a woman I had just met. I had told her about the death sentence my doctors had given me and she had told me about Aboriginal healers. And here I was, alone in Australia, dialing a number that was my only link to those healers. A number that no one was answering.

My heart sank as I heard the ringing stop and an answering machine pick up. But then I heard Ray's now-familiar voice saying, "Hi Gary," and I breathed a sigh of relief. He had left a recording for me on his answering machine. He told me there was a reservation at a nearby hotel under my name and that once I'd had a chance to rest, he'd contact me. The message ended with: "By the way, Mate, welcome to Australia."

I was so tired I could hardly wheel myself to the taxi stand. At the hotel registration desk that night, I had so little control over my hands that I could only manage a shaky *X* for a signature. Finally, I was in my room. I stretched out on the bed, fully clothed, and immediately fell into an exhausted sleep.

Just after 9:00 a.m. I awoke to a knocking at the door. "Hey, Mate. It's Ray. Are you ready to go?"

"I'm just getting up," I responded as I fumbled my way out of bed.

"Okay. We'll go along in a minute."

I don't know what I expected, but Ray was a wonderful surprise. He had been terse, almost rude, when I had first called about coming to Australia. Now, as I opened the door, the grin he flashed me was like a mischievous little boy's. Dressed in khaki shorts and a brightly colored sports shirt, Ray was average in height and weight, with light brown skin and a tousled mass of silvery-gray hair. One eye socket was closed over an injured eye, and his shirtsleeve revealed the stump of his right arm. He appeared to be in his late forties. For some reason I felt a powerful and immediate connection, as if I'd known him for a very long time.

After a quick stop at Ray's apartment, we made our way through Brisbane, past densely packed buildings and apartment complexes much like any city in the States. I saw no sign of overt poverty, though Ray let me know that many Aboriginal people who had relocated to Australia's cities struggled to make a living. Within fifteen minutes of leaving the outskirts, we were driving through an open, bare countryside of nothing but rock and sand. The sun and heat were fierce, beating down on the car.

We approached a river, the only sign of moisture in this parched landscape. Sunlight shimmering over the ripples lifted my spirits, as I'd always loved water and had been a competitive marathon swimmer.

Ray glanced over at me and tilted his head toward the river as the road swung away from it. "Say good-bye to the world as you once knew it."

I turned my neck as best I could for a last glimpse of the beautiful river, my mood plummeting as abruptly as it had risen. Did Ray mean I should say good-bye to life? To water and food, to my children and everything I had loved? Was this journey only about accepting my imminent death? At that moment I had no idea what lay ahead for me in Ray's tribal village. Several weeks later, returning over this road past the same river, I would realize that he'd been telling me to say good-bye to my old belief system and the way of life that was killing me.

The farther we went into the Outback, the worse the roads became. We were soon following a badly paved, one-lane asphalt road, the ride bumpy and dusty. The last sign of "civilization" was a shack sitting by itself at the side of the road. Ray pulled right up to its window and ordered hamburgers at this Outback equivalent of a drive-in, our last chance to eat and drink before the remaining six- or seven-hour drive to his village. I was ravenous, after no dinner or breakfast, so eagerly bit into the meat patty between slices of white bread with no condiments.

Ray took a bite and nodded in approval. "As usual."

It wasn't until days later that Ray, under duress, confessed to the real identity of that unique-tasting burger. It didn't come from a cow. Cows are scarce in Australia. It was crocodile.

After eating, we drove further into the baking desert. Around three in the afternoon, thirsty and gritty with dust, I asked Ray how far we still had to go.

"Not far," he answered. "Believe me, Mate, this is a short drive by Australian standards. Now, if we were going to Perth, it would take us a good week's worth of driving. Be patient. We could be going on a walkabout, you know." He grinned.

Finally, at around 9:00 p.m., Ray announced, "Here we are." He turned off the rough main highway onto an even rougher dirt access road. "There's the village."

At first I didn't see a thing, even though the moon was bright. Then gradually, at about twenty-five yards' distance, a village of a dozen or so small huts seemed to slowly emerge from the landscape. Every building, every object blended perfectly into its surroundings. As best I could see, the thatched houses were made of wood scraps, twigs, and leaves. There were a couple of people moving about in the shadows, but no one came over to the car, and I was too exhausted to care.

As Ray helped me out of the car and into my wheelchair, the effects of my two-day journey from America to Australia suddenly caught up with me. I could hardly move. After wheeling me to a dirt-floored hut with uncurtained openings for windows, Ray asked, "Do you need any help?"

"No, I'll be okay." All I could think about was lying down. As soon as he was gone, I eased my way out of my wheelchair onto the "bed"—a plain wooden plank. Using my knapsack as a pillow, I fell, for the second night in a row, into the total oblivion of exhausted sleep. I slept for eleven hours straight and did not awaken until midmorning of the next day.

When I awoke, groggy after so much sleep, I had a moment of sheer disorientation as to where I was. My back hurt, and I had a kink in my neck from the hard surface I was lying on. The rough wood of the walls and ceiling didn't look like any bedroom I'd ever known.

A moment later it all came back to me. I was in the Outback, and the voices outside my hut speaking in a language I had never heard before were honest-to-god Aboriginal people. I felt a surge of excitement.

Heaving myself into my chair, I took stock of my surroundings. The bed I had spent the night on consisted of a pair of tree stumps holding a narrow wooden sleeping platform a couple of feet above a dirt floor. To the side stood a taller and wider stump that I surmised was a table. Everything was as bare and utilitarian as possible. There was no bedding, not even a blanket, no attached door, and no glass in the window openings.

Hoping to see Ray, I wheeled myself outside. I squinted in the glaring sunlight, the sun already climbing above a reddish dust haze and cooking the flat landscape. I would soon learn that even at night, the temperatures here rarely dipped below 90 degrees, and could reach 130 during the day. The bare vista of sand and rocks was relieved only by a few trees dotting the horizon.

My guide was nowhere in sight, but the villagers, about twenty Aboriginal people of varying ages, were awake and going about their daily routines. On average the men were about 5' 3" and the women about 4' 11". Everyone was barefoot, and some of the smaller children were naked. The men were dressed in loincloths and most of them were clean shaven, but some had facial hair that was extremely coarse and curly. The women wore simple skirts or shifts, a few going bare breasted. No one wore jewelry or any type of decoration.

I was surprised by the variety of skin colors, which varied from light brown to the deepest black. This evidence of their mixed blood reminded me of what Ray had told me about the history of his people during our long car trip. Because of the legacy of rape, "pacification," and intermarriage, the Aboriginal people were now all the colors of the rainbow.

The adults glanced discreetly in my direction, while the children openly stared. Soon some of the younger ones began to play tag with one another, circling closer and closer to my wheelchair. When a child got too close, he or she would run away, shrieking with laughter, only to return a few minutes later. Some of the adults and teenagers smiled and spoke to me in their own language as they walked past.

In spite of the shy friendliness that the villagers displayed toward me, I could not shake the uncomfortable feeling that I was an intruder into someone else's private world. It's hard to be somewhere where you don't understand the language and have nothing to contribute. Everyone seemed to have a purpose but me, the scruffy-looking white guy with the two-day growth of beard. Next to the small graceful shapes of the villagers, I felt large and ungainly, even seated in my wheelchair.

Finally I was unable to stand the strangeness any longer, and I wheeled myself back into the safety of my hut. I found myself saying a little prayer: "It's up to you now, God. I'm here, but I am totally out of control. I'm in a strange land surrounded by unfamiliar people living a life I don't understand. Just help me get through this day."

A few minutes later a middle-aged woman dressed in a long, loose skirt and a blouse appeared at the door of my hut, bringing me a gourd filled with water and a kind of "muffin" in a wooden bowl. It was hard to tell how old she was, but I thought she might be about Ray's age, in her mid-forties. She was the healer he had told me about.

I'm not sure what I expected—perhaps some mysterious

indigenous-looking person wearing amulets, muttering spells over me. Instead, Rose was a gentle and dignified woman who greeted me in perfect English with a British accent. Her thick brown hair, peppered with gray, was pulled back off her face, and her tanned-looking skin had deep lines etched in it from the sun. When she smiled, however, her whole appearance softened.

"Welcome," she exclaimed. "I heard you were awake. I'm Rose, the healer you will be working with for most of your stay with us. I'm sure you've had a difficult time, but the journey you're beginning right now will be a rewarding one."

Rose told me that everyone in the village had been looking forward to my arrival. "We've spent four months getting ready for you," she disclosed. "Now that you are here, we are all overjoyed to see you. We've been waiting a long time."

This comment took me by surprise. "Wait a minute," I protested. "Four months ago I didn't know I'd be coming here. In fact, I didn't even know how sick I was back then. I only knew I was coming here about two weeks ago. What do you mean, you knew I was coming?"

"The Big Guy told us."

"Who's the 'Big Guy'?"

Rose smiled. "I guess you would call him 'God,' but to us he is simply everything that is."

She could see that I was struggling with this concept, not only of a god that was "everything that is" but also that the tribe knew I was coming before I did. However, she didn't enlighten me further. She simply changed the subject, explaining why the village had chosen Ray and her to work with me. It was because they could help bridge the gap between my world and the world of the traditional Aboriginal people.

"Ray has lived in Brisbane off and on for many years," she informed me. "He's still a member of the tribe, but he knows a great deal about the white world. His children and grandchildren are trying to live in it, and he is a good man who will not abandon them or allow them to forget their heritage.

"I have lived in both worlds also. My mother was an Aborigine and my father was white. I learned to speak fluent English when I was very young and was educated in Brisbane, where my mother and I lived for years."

Rose indicated she and Ray had worked together to find ways to communicate concepts of Aboriginal medicine to me. "We have spent a lot of time thinking about the metaphors that would be meaningful to someone from your culture. Sometimes we will be asking you to think in our metaphors, but much of the time we will try to speak to you in terms you can understand."

I didn't entirely understand what she meant by "meaningful metaphors," but I was ready to move forward. I asked Rose when we would begin my treatment. She advised that I should rest for the remainder of the day. The next morning Ray would come by and wheel me down to her treatment room on the outskirts of the village.

I slept for another four hours that afternoon, waking at sunset. Pulling myself into my wheelchair, I rolled over to the doorway to see what was going on. The village was stirring, people moving between huts.

"Evening, Mate. Thought you might sleep through it." It was Ray, ambling over from a nearby hut.

"Sleep through what?"

"Your welcome celebration. Come on." Ray pushed me forward over the packed dirt toward the gathering. In the dusk some men were tending a fire in a rock-lined pit in the middle of an open area.

By our standards there wasn't much sign of festivity, though some of the men who'd earlier gone about naked were now wearing gourds to cover their privates, and a few of the women had donned plain, loose blouses and skirts. The five or six children of the village were still running around naked, playing, but I noticed a general quiet that surprised me. The kids didn't do much of the usual shrieking and shouting, nor the adults the chatting that would mark a social occasion in my own cultural experience. Later I would learn from Ray and Rose that the Aboriginal tribe's people communicated mostly through telepathy, so they didn't really need to speak aloud.

Ray wheeled me over to a spot on the periphery of the gathering circle, where the women were setting out cooked meats, fruit, and tuber-like vegetables. Before we ate, I was formally welcomed and honored by each of the villagers. One by one the people came up to greet me. Most of the men hugged me. Although I came from a culture, a family, and a business world where men did not express their feelings in this way, I felt quite comfortable and "comforted" by the sincerity of their embrace.

The women did not hug me, but when I held out my hand to shake theirs, each one of them grasped me by my index finger, smiled, and uttered some words of greeting. Although I was the only white person there, I didn't feel as if any of them were looking at my skin color, but rather at my heart. When people gave me their names, Ray told me not to worry about remembering all of them. I couldn't even if I'd tried, because they all sounded to me like guttural sounds of three or four syllables.

Finally, everyone sat down on the ground to eat. The villagers piled their food on large leaves and ate with their fingers, but a woman brought me my food in a wooden bowl. I was a little nervous about eating things I couldn't identify, but everything was surprisingly tasty.

Ray told me the meat was wild boar some of the men had brought back from a hunt. Usually dinner was a vegetable or fruit and grubs or insects. I was very hungry, and the meat tasted delicious. As I thought this, I glanced up to see the woman who had brought it to me beaming at me across the circle and nodding. Beside her, an old man with a very dark, wrinkled face and a wild bird's nest of gray hair and beard sat watching me, unblinking. Ordinarily, such a penetrating gaze would have made me uncomfortable, but somehow this didn't bother me.

It was a very leisurely gathering, people eating slowly, occasionally saying something. After an hour or two they started chanting and singing. One man brought out what looked like a crooked branch, and I recognized it as a didgeridoo, after seeing one in Ray's apartment. I had asked Ray then if he would play it for me, but he'd told me it was someone else's, and only the person it was made for could play it.

The haunting, eerie sounds of the wind instrument filled the night, and I sat in a strangely peaceful spell, watching the flames as a few of the men and women got up to move around in a free-form dance. Part of me felt lonely, an alien in the midst of this foreign gathering, locked in my wheelchair and my ignorance of these people's language. But another part of me felt oddly connected in a way I couldn't understand.

A state of profound stillness and peace filled me. In the firelight the people and my surroundings soon took on an almost magical aspect. Gradually, I became aware that I was seeing a glowing envelope of light around each person. I looked away, squeezed my eyes shut, then opened them and blinked a couple of times. When I looked back at the villagers, everyone was still glowing.

"What's the matter?" Ray asked.

"I don't know quite how to say this, but I'm seeing rings of light around everyone," I confided. "My eyes must be playing tricks on me."

"There's nothing wrong with your eyes, Mate. You're just seeing their energy. In your culture you'd call it their auras."

Ray put his hand companionably on my shoulder. "It's nothing to be afraid of. Because you're out here you're beginning to understand some of our ways, that's all. It kind of rubs off on you. Before you leave you'll be able to see a lot of things. You don't know it yet, but you have many gifts, and we're going to show you how to use some of them. Over time you'll learn to use others on your own. They'll just evolve."

I didn't really understand what he was telling me, but in my peaceful state with my full belly, I let it pass. I was content and, oddly, I didn't feel afraid anymore. As the embers died down I glanced across the circle to see the grizzled old man watching me again. I smiled and he nodded.

The next morning I awoke rested and eager to get started.

Ray popped his head in through the open doorway. "Ready, Mate?"

I told him I could manage my chair, but he insisted on pushing me. I was already learning that it was useless arguing with him, so I let him steer me along the dirt path. We made quite the pair—a man with one arm and one eye, maneuvering the crippled man in a wheelchair toward an old shanty in the middle of the Outback of Australia, where miracles would be performed.

Back home I had been surrounded with the finest doctors, medical equipment, and facilities money could buy. Now I found myself in a wooden hut approximately eight feet square with a dirt floor and a small painted chair. Rose was sitting in the chair waiting for me. I realized then that I hadn't seen her at the gathering the night before, and I wondered why her healing hut was set at a distance from the rest of the villagers.

Once again I had expected something different—a room filled with bunches of drying herbs hanging from the rafters and tinctures in clay pots sitting on rows of shelves along the wall. I had no idea what we would be able to accomplish in this stark setting.

Ray turned to go.

"Aren't you going to stay with me?" I called after him.

"No, Mate. The first few days you'll only be workin' with Rose. I'll be back to get you tonight."

I watched with some trepidation as he walked away. But Rose's smile put me at ease, and I was eager to begin whatever we were going to do in this "treatment room."

"So what's next?" I asked. "Where do we begin?"

"Today we're going to do a lot of talking, and you're going to do most of it," Rose stated in her pleasant British accent. She clarified that she couldn't begin treating me until she knew a lot more about me and until I knew a lot more about the basic premises behind Aboriginal healing.

"If you are to get well and stay well, Gary, you will have to transform from the inside out. We'll start by finding out which experiences and beliefs generated your MS."

Beliefs and experiences? Wait a minute. Although no one knew what caused MS, I was quite sure it had nothing to do with beliefs and experiences.

"What do you mean, 'the experiences and beliefs that created my MS'?"

"There is a connection between your illness and the rest of your life," Rose replied. "We are going to address the roots of your illness, unlike Western medicine, which only treats the outward symptoms, leaving the body to fight the cause of the illness unassisted."

I wasn't convinced. My mind was grappling to make logical connections between the primitive music with dancing around the fire last night and this non-native-looking woman, sitting rather primly, analyzing my illness in her British accent. But all I could do was surrender to the incongruities, so I relented, "Okay, I'm listening."

"Well," reasoned Rose, "if you had a dandelion weed growing in an undesirable place, you would want to get rid of it before it spread or did damage. But if you merely cut off the top of the plant, thinking this would kill it, it would keep on returning. Unless the root is pulled out, the weed will continue to thrive.

"That is what happens within our own bodies. The root of an illness, where it all began, is what carries its power, not the symptoms. When my people talk about healing, we include not only the body, but also the mind, emotions, and spirit."

Rose explained that in our first few sessions, I would need to tell her my story so that she could see where the roots of MS had taken hold. She wanted to know about my first experience of MS, what I was doing at the time, what my life was like, how I reacted to my illness, and what had happened since then.

I still wasn't convinced, but here I was, thousands of miles from home, risking it all on the chance that this woman knew something that I (and my Western doctors) didn't. And so I told her my story, from that day when my foot began to drag, to a chance encounter in a jazz club that started me on a trip to the Australian Outback.

As I talked Rose listened with interest and compassion. I could see no sign of pity.

As I wound my story up she leaned forward and touched my hand. "Gary, you've been through a lot. I want you to know that our medicine can heal you."

She let that sink in. Then she added, "But you will have to let go of a lot of your preconceptions before that can happen. Everything you have seen about doctoring in the U.S. is based on science and logic. Our medicine might not seem logical to you, but we do have our own kind of "science." While you are here with us, you will be reaching into the depths of your spirit to find the answers about why you are sick and what you need to do to become well."

"What makes you think I can do that?" I asked.

Rose smiled. "We've already seen you walking," she asserted.

Despite my skepticism, my heart leaped in hope. She had already seen me walking! As we broke for lunch that thought reverberated in my mind.

When I was told that I had only two years to live, the thought had repeated in my head like a broken record: *Two years. Two years. Two years.* But now I had a new recording, one that I was happy to hear: *We have seen you walking. We have seen you walking.*

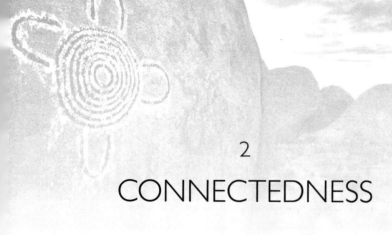

2
CONNECTEDNESS

After a break for lunch Rose was ready to continue our session, but I still didn't see why I needed to tell her so much about my life. "I just want to get healed of MS. And I really don't see what my history has to do with it."

Rose smoothed her drab skirt over her knees as she studied my face. Finally she asked, "Have you ever squeezed an orange? What did you get? Orange juice, of course. The only thing that will come out of the orange is what's already inside.

"And human beings are the same. So, therefore, our first step is to find out what is inside you and why you have chosen multiple sclerosis."

I was taken aback. It was one thing when she referred to experiences and beliefs that caused my MS. But now to say it was a choice? The very idea made me angry. It was a ludicrous thought, a sort of "blaming-the-victim-for-the-crime" mentality, and I wanted nothing to do with it.

"Wait a minute. Are you telling me that I *caused* my multiple sclerosis?"

"I know this is a difficult concept for you to understand," Rose acknowledged. "But this has nothing to do with blame. Blame is only a negative step backward. What we are talking about here is learning to take responsibility for everything that happens to us. That is a positive step forward. Nothing in our life ever changes until we realize we have choices.

"Whether you know it or not, your MS is a chosen condition," she continued. "You will come to understand this later. If you feel angry, that's all right, because anger is a normal mechanism that helps us to survive in our physical world."

She still didn't have me convinced. There was no way I would have chosen this miserable illness. Why would anyone choose to be sick? Illness was always the luck of the draw. I was just one of the unlucky ones. Multiple sclerosis had nothing to do with my "inner self" or any of that New Age babble. Everyone knew that illness was caused by bacteria, or by a part of the body that broke down and stopped functioning. A virus caused a cold. A cancer cell caused cancer. A nonfunctioning pancreas caused diabetes. Plugged arteries caused heart attacks.

My hands gripped the wheels of my chair, ready to take me away from this nonsense. But even as the arguments were piling up in my mind, I could see my "facts" beginning to evaporate. Which of these illnesses had modern medical science actually cured? We could control and treat the symptoms, but had we ever learned to eradicate the disease?

And when people suffered from identical illnesses and received identical treatments, why did some people recover and others die? Why would one person exposed to a virus become ill, and another remain well? Could there be other factors underlying illness, beyond just the physical? My physicist's mind forced me to agree that this might be so. I was going to have to listen to what Rose proposed with an open mind.

I forced my hands to relax and took a deep breath. "I'm not saying that I'm agreeing with you," I contended, "but if I chose to have MS, how did that happen? Did I just wake up one morning and decide to get sick? I didn't even know what MS was! So how could I possibly choose it?"

"Through the power of your own thoughts and emotions, Gary." Rose had been waiting patiently. "The Aboriginal people believe that a person's mind exists in every part of his body, in every single cell. Because of this, every thought we have, each emotion we experience, has a physical effect upon our body.

"Think about this for a moment. Can you create a thought that makes you sick? People do it every day. Stress causes both physical and emotional maladies. When you worry about a problem you are having, you can give yourself a headache. Or you can become so upset about something that you begin to feel nauseous and shaky, and can even cause yourself to vomit."

I had to concur I could see the connection between stress and an upset stomach or a headache. But MS?

Rose smiled as if she could read my thoughts. "Not only are we affected by our *conscious* thoughts, but by our *subconscious* ones as well," she continued. "My people believe that there is an intelligence behind our thoughts that creates the chemical reactions within our bodies. If you were to ask me what comes first, the thought or the physical manifestation, I would say it's the thought."

I was sure she could see in my face the struggle I was having with what she was saying.

"Okay," she said. "This is why the tribe had Ray bring me here to work with you, even though I don't belong to this village, because I grew up and worked in the white man's world. I was just as skeptical as you are when I first returned to my own people, just as caught up in logic. So let's talk in your language for a while, the language of a physicist. Scientists have discovered that in the nervous system there is an incoming signal, a new pulse, every time we feel something. And every time there's a new thought, a new emotion, your neurotransmitters send messages throughout your entire body."

I nodded in agreement.

"These messages latch on to neuroreceptors, which are attached to every single cell. Depending on the nature of the new thought or the new emotion, these transmitters will latch on to specific types of receptors rather than others. That's why certain emotions and thoughts will create certain conditions in your body."

"Well," I insisted, "I know that I have no sense of feeling in my body with my MS. My receptors are shut down. There's scar tissue around them instead of myelin. But what does this have to do with choice?" I couldn't seem to let go of my outrage over that notion.

"The connection is that, a long time ago, you chose to stop feeling your emotions," Rose explained. "If you accept what I've said about thoughts manifesting physically, then you will see that you've created a parallel situation in your body. Physically, you are numb and unable to move. That's what the nervous system is all about—feeling."

I had to admit that hit home. If there was anything in the universe that I was incompetent at, it was dealing with feelings. But could there really be a connection between that and this horrible disease?

Rose smiled at me reassuringly, the creases of her weathered face softening. "Gary, it's all going to make sense in a bit. Right now, I want you to tell me more about your life. I know when your body became numb. Now I want you to tell me about when your spirit became numb—when you stopped yourself from feeling. There's no hurry, no need to tie it all together. Just talk about whatever comes up."

Somehow I trusted her. So I let my mind drift, thinking about how and why I had learned to keep a tight lid on my feelings. Immediately, I thought of my alcoholic father, who vented his rage on everyone in the family through physical and verbal abuse.

I told Rose about him, about how I learned to keep quiet around him and disappear as quickly as possible. It was a skill that I learned well and practiced often, because it was a matter of survival around my father. I knew that his rages and beatings would be inflicted only upon the one unwise enough to speak out or unfortunate enough to be within arm's length. Although my mother was a kind woman, she was powerless to stand up to my dad.

After one too many beatings during which my mother watched helplessly, I decided that I could depend on no one but myself. I had to take life into my own hands. As far as I was concerned, I had no parents.

I told Rose how sports became a haven away from my family, a place where I got my first real taste of praise. I was a natural athlete, and whatever the season, I was involved, whether it was baseball, football, basketball, ice hockey, or bowling. There were countless hours, year-round, spent in the bowling alley, doing homework in the locker room and just hanging out.

I also found refuge in the world of facts and logic, for I excelled in math and science. One day my eighth-grade teacher wrote down an algebraic formula on the blackboard. It looked like a series of codes, a puzzle to decipher, and I was intrigued by the challenge it presented. My mind worked quickly, and I suddenly knew the answer. Excitement ran through me like a jolt of electricity. I was hooked on the world of the mind.

I'd found a home where I could finally feel safe—in my head and away from my heart. When I was given achievement tests in school, my scores in math and science were always in the top percentiles. Because my father constantly ridiculed me, telling me that I was stupid, this validation that I was smart was extremely important to me.

I liked the world of science. It made sense to me. In science there are certain set material laws that govern our world. The speed of light is invariable; gravity and the laws of trajectory never fail us. There is a physical order to every life process and a principle behind it. I decided that hard, cold facts, the scientific method, and the process of logical reasoning were the real foundations for true knowledge.

"These beliefs gave me an escape from the family problems I could not solve," I told Rose. "They became the essence of all I knew to be true. I didn't have to feel. I could just think."

After high school I found another way to escape from the pain of my family. I joined the Army, where I was trained in electronics. After the Army I studied physics in college and then joined the Coast Guard, where I continued to study electronics. I eventually started my own company, Holz Industries, and became very successful in the scientific field, designing microwave components for land, sea, and air.

"And that's my story," I finished. "The world of science has been good to me. It's a world I understand and can operate in."

"Yes," Rose agreed. "It sounds like you were pretty successful in your career. But I haven't heard you mention relationships." She raised an eyebrow. "Did you have friends? Girlfriends? Did you marry? Have children? Tell me about that."

I gave a long sigh. This was not a story I enjoyed telling. But Rose was waiting patiently, hands folded in her lap, clearly not about to move until I'd told it all.

"Well, my attempts at relationships were not so successful," I finally began. "I knew something was missing, and somewhere along the way, I decided that I could fix it if I could just somehow acquire all the outward appearances of an ordinary life. That was the belief that propelled me into my first marriage."

It all started the Christmas when I had just returned from a fifteen-month assignment in Korea. I met Harry, a musician playing at a local hangout across from Fort Campbell, and he invited me to his parents' home for Christmas dinner. When we drove up to their red brick ranch house at the edge of town, there were patches of snow beneath the barren trees, and fragrant wood smoke rose from the fireplace. Inside, the smell of baking corn bread and simmering white beans filled my senses, and the lights from the Christmas tree cast a warm glow over everything. Harry's mom, dad, and sister, Sue, were all kind and welcoming. I was immediately attracted to Sue, who was very pretty, with large brown eyes, a sweet smile, and a soft Southern drawl.

This friendliness and warmth was a new experience for me, and I quickly fell in love with the idea of a real family. Not surprisingly, after a year of dating, Sue and I were married.

But the marriage was in trouble almost from the start. We struggled to establish communication and intimacy. We broke up and made up. We had two beautiful children, and at times we appeared to be a loving family. But I had been so obsessed with getting love that I had never learned how to give it. It was a struggle to attain any level of real intimacy with my wife.

When I tried to talk about this with Sue, I only managed to damage our relationship further. What I was attempting to say was that I felt inept in loving her and my children and was trying to find my way. She thought I was saying I didn't love her.

Shortly thereafter I was served divorce papers. I took the path of least resistance and chose not to fight the divorce. When I returned home from a business trip a few weeks later, I opened the door to an empty house. My children, then one year old and three years old, had been taken out of state with their mother to live with her parents. As I stood in that empty house, I saw that I had come full circle, back to where I had begun. The family I'd longed for and tried to create had totally disappeared.

I agreed to give Sue custody of our children because I believed that I was incapable of caring for them. They needed to be with their mother, and she needed to be with her family. I knew that my in-laws would provide a good home for Sue and the children. That home just wouldn't include me. I convinced myself that it was the best solution.

I do not remember making a conscious choice not to see my children, but that is what I did. The years passed, and the contact between us dwindled. Perhaps I just couldn't risk the pain of being rejected. It was easier to go numb. I paid child support, sent birthday cards, bought Christmas gifts. But I rarely saw my son and daughter; although, they were often in my thoughts. I believed they were better off without me.

That's when I met Tina. She was my exact opposite—passionate, vivacious, and talkative. And she shared my love for ballroom dancing. I thought it was a good match. We would balance each other out. I was happy that I had been given a second chance to create the family I wanted.

For the first three months of our marriage, we were pretty happy. But eventually our differences became a source of conflict. Tina's Italian family had taught her to express her emotions freely and to argue with gusto. My dysfunctional family had taught me to avoid conflict—to keep quiet and, as soon as possible, to disappear. The result was total disaster.

We started seeing a counselor, but our marriage continued to deteriorate. Tina would try to goad me into being emotionally responsive, but the more she shouted, the more I withdrew. At the time I didn't think I was the one with the problem. If only my wife could get fixed, then our marriage would be okay. So we limped on, each of us alone in our individual pain. I continued to numb myself to the whole situation and kept my attention on my business.

"I see." Rose had been sitting motionless in her wooden chair as I told her about these events in my life. Now she leaned forward. "You learned how to become emotionally numb as a survival skill around your father. By the time you married and had children, it was too engrained to let go of it. Is that it?"

I slowly nodded. "It didn't seem like I had a choice," I replied. "It just seemed like that's the way I was, and I didn't know how to be different."

"Did anything change when you were diagnosed with MS?" she asked. "Sometimes a serious illness can be a wake-up call that forces us to change."

"Actually, I did try to change," I told her. "I tried to heal the relationship with my children. Suddenly the idea of never seeing my children again became worse than the thought of dying. When I received an invitation to attend a business conference in Tennessee, near where they lived, I made the decision to go and see them. I wanted to build some kind of relationship with them before it was too late. They were about thirteen and fifteen then."

"How did that go?" Rose inquired.

"Not well," I admitted. "In fact, it was terrible."

Tina had gone with me on the visit, and we were greeted at the door by Sue's parents. Sue was not there. So we sat down with them in the living room and proceeded to make polite small talk.

Eventually my daughter and son appeared and sat down. They were scared to death. My son was completely emotionally detached from the situation, and my daughter seemed very uneasy. My former in-laws, who clearly disliked me underneath all their politeness, never left me alone with the children. The whole situation was very strained. I was clearly an outsider to the family I had once been a part of.

Tina and I stayed for only half an hour. As we drove away, I felt like a failure. My children were almost grown up, and I had missed sharing most of their lives. I was flooded with memories. When my daughter was a baby, I had been the center of her universe. I remembered holding and rocking her when she was crying from cutting teeth. I remembered the joy I felt when I saw my son for the first time in the hospital delivery room, and how I had cried when I held him. How had I ever allowed myself to let go of my children? I just couldn't understand it. What I had lost was immense, and the loss cut deep.

The only real intimacy I had ever known had been in my relationship with my children when they were young. And now they seemed afraid of me! I could clearly see that they had no idea who I was or why I had left their lives. What scared me most of all was the knowledge that I had inadvertently repeated my own father's abandonment of me. My children were suffering from the physical absence of their father just as I had suffered from the emotional absence of mine. The words of Harry Chapin's song, "Cat's in the Cradle," kept playing in my head. Without meaning to, I had grown up to be like my dad.

My story drew to a close as the sun was going down, casting an ironically rosy light through the open window and doorway cut into the rough wood wall. Sweat prickled on my face and back, and I suddenly realized how hot and stuffy the room was, no breeze stirring outside or in.

Rose sat quietly for a few moments, hands in her lap. Then she said, "Thank you for sharing this with me, Gary. I know it has been painful to revisit these old memories, but it's necessary for me to know about your life in order to create the right program for your healing."

She paused, and then added, "And I know that you're still resisting seeing a connection between your emotional numbness and your MS, but just keep your mind open."

"All right."

"Good." The voice came from behind me.

I startled, turning my wheelchair to see Ray looking in through one of the window gaps. "Time for dinner, Mate."

"See you in the morning, Gary," Rose called, as Ray started to push me out of the hut.

"Wait." I put my hand on a wheel, stopping the chair. "Aren't you coming to dinner?"

She hesitated, and a look passed between her and Ray, "I'm not a member of this tribe, Gary. I stay in the visitor hut." She indicated the other small hut behind the healing room, both of them set aside from the nearby cluster of the village.

I was confused, but decided it wasn't my place to question why I was allowed to eat and sleep with the tribe. Ray didn't elaborate as he pushed me toward my hut, just left me there with a brief, "I'll bring us some grub."

I hadn't realized Ray meant that literally, but when he returned with two wooden bowls, I realized that in addition to a baked root of some kind, the main course was indeed grubs. And they were still wriggling.

I stalled by eating the vegetable and drinking the warm water from a gourd, while I watched Ray pop the fat grubs into his mouth with apparent relish. He was watching me with a glint in his one good eye, and I dreaded his wicked sense of humor more than I did the meal. I popped one into my mouth, intending to swallow it whole, and then realized he was waiting to see me chew. It actually didn't taste that bad. And I knew I'd need my strength for the work to come, so I finished them off.

Ray took my bowl with a chuckle, and then settled back against the rough wall, shirtless in his loose shorts. He rubbed the stump of his arm, a habit I'd observed earlier. "Well, Mate, how'd it go today?"

That set the pattern for most of my time to come—working with Rose during the day, and then eating and talking it over with Ray in the evening. Occasionally there would be a village gathering, for a celebration or when the hunters brought some meat home, but mostly I would eat in my own hut.

That night I was having trouble with the whole idea that my history was connected to my disease, so Ray told me more about the Aboriginal theory of connectedness. He explained they have a word for it that roughly translates as "environment," but includes everything inside a person as well as everything outside—inner and outer environment.

"We are connected not just to each other and to the world that we live in, but our body, mind, and soul are connected, inseparable," he related. "In the West, you think of your environment as being something outside of you, but the truth is, you *are* your environment."

I just shook my head, confused.

Ray looked at me quizzically. "Tell me, Mate, what makes up a human being?"

"Well," I held up a finger. "I have a body . . ."

"That's right."

" . . . and a mind." I held up another finger. "And a soul."

Ray took hold of my three fingers and squeezed them together. "Look, Mate, this is what is really happening inside of you. In your culture you spend a lot of time going to seminars and reading books about integrating your body, mind, and soul. The truth is, they were never separate. From the day you were born, you were a body-mind-soul. What you do to one has a direct effect on the others *because they are one and the same thing.*"

He grinned. "Add to that the fact that we are never separate from the environment around us. The winds, the rain, the soil, they all affect us and we affect them. When it's going to rain, you can feel it inside. You get tense and feel like something is about to happen. When the rains fall, you feel relieved and refreshed."

Letting go of my fingers, Ray leaned back and studied me with his usual impassive expression that had fooled me before I saw his underlying humor and warmth. "It's all your environment, Gary. If your internal and external universe are working in harmony, you will be healthy spiritually and physically. If you create an external environment that isn't healthy, you won't be able to maintain any internal healing. So, Mate, your *physical* condition is directly related to your *spiritual* condition. And that is up to you."

That night I lay on my hard bed and pondered the matter of connectedness. Could there really be a connection between all the events of my life, the decisions that I had made, the beliefs that I had adopted— and my illness, multiple sclerosis?

I thought I escaped my dismal childhood and my father's legacy.

Could it be that my father's inability to face his demons had now become mine? I didn't use a bottle to numb myself, but my ability to shut off my emotions worked just as well. And now my whole body was going numb. Perhaps this disease was simply mirroring the emotional numbness I had experienced for a long time. Perhaps it was mirroring in my body what had already happened in my spirit.

These thoughts began to create cracks in my world view about what makes people healthy and what makes them sick. It was depressing to think that I had not only numbed myself to life, but perhaps numbed my body as well. But I also felt a glimmer of hope.

Before, my MS had seemed like some dreadful misfortune that had come into my life and mysteriously struck me down. But if there were emotional, mental, and spiritual "reasons" for my body shutting down, then perhaps I might be able to undo some of the damage and at least keep myself from dying.

As I lay there waiting for sleep, I felt very small and alone in my flimsy hut beneath the vastness of the night sky. I could sense the desolate stretches of the Outback all around me, offering little comfort. All I could do was hold to the fragile hope Rose and Ray were offering—that somehow I held the key to my own healing.

3

WILLINGNESS

Despite the night's fears, I slept well on my hard bed and awoke the next morning eager to continue with my treatment. After pulling myself into my chair, I peered out at the sun already baking the red dirt.

I was surprised to see what looked like most of the villagers standing or sitting outside my hut, their eyes fixed on me. They weren't talking, and the kids weren't playing—they just seemed to be waiting for my appearance. I raised a hand and called out, "Good morning."

No reaction. At a loss, I looked around and was relieved to see Ray ambling over with my breakfast in a wooden bowl. He murmured something to the group and came into the hut with me as the others went their ways.

"Afraid you're the main event, Mate," he commented. "Most of them haven't seen too many white men, and they're curious about your wheelchair."

Again, I felt like an alien and wished I could at least speak to the others a little. But their language was no more than baffling sounds to me, and from the hints I was getting from Ray and Rose, it seemed like spoken words were only a small part of the way they communicated, anyway.

As soon as I'd finished my muffinlike breakfast, we were off to see Rose. She greeted me with her usual pleasant smile and told me we were going to spend some time looking at the Five Essentials of Healing.

Hearing this, I felt a little impatient. I wanted to get on with the "real" healing. After all, the clock was ticking. When you've been told that you have only two years to live, days are not given up lightly.

Rose shook her head slightly. "I know you feel a sense of urgency, Gary, but this is a vital part of the healing process. What we're doing is building a foundation. I told you that Aboriginal healing has a spiritual basis, and there are some concepts that you've got to understand before we can proceed."

"Okay," I resigned. "Tell me about these essentials."

"We talked yesterday about connectedness. You might think of it as the mortar that holds the whole system together. But now we have to put some bricks in place that will become the foundation for the deeper and more specific healing that we do. There are five bricks, the Five Essentials of Healing." She held up her hand and ticked them off. "They are Willingness, Awareness, Acceptance, Empowerment, and Focus."

"So we're going to be laying bricks this morning," I joked. "It sounds like a lot of hard work. Are you sure I'm up to it?"

"That's entirely up to you," Rose answered seriously. "In fact, that's the first question that I want you to ask yourself. The most important prerequisite to getting well is really wanting to, subconsciously as well as consciously. Willingness is the key that unlocks the door to health. It is the first Essential of Healing. So, Gary, are you willing to get well?"

I was astonished that she would even ask. "Of course, I'm willing. I'm here, aren't I?"

"Well, we'll see." She gave me a mysterious smile. "Most of us on a conscious level want to be healed. However, on a subconscious level, we may not feel the same. We may have a hidden agenda buried within. There is often a resistance and an unwillingness to change, because change runs against the typical human mindset.

"You need to be willing, on all levels of consciousness, for change to take place so healing can begin. A great deal of our initial work will be in testing your belief system and finding what is really true for you on a subconscious level. You will find that in many areas you are sabotaging yourself."

"Well, that may be true about some things, but I know for a fact that I'm willing to get well," I responded. "You have no idea what I've gone through to get here. It's been an incredible journey."

"Why don't you tell me about it, Gary?" Rose answered. "I know that you met Carolyn, who put you in contact with Ray. And that Ray brought you out here to work with us. But tell me how that all came about and why you trusted the two of them enough to travel thousands of miles and put yourself in our hands."

Why had I trusted them? It was a good question, one I didn't know the answer to. But I could at least tell Rose how the whole thing had happened.

"It all started with a chance encounter in a jazz club," I told her. "I had gone there to see if I could escape for a while. After I was told that I had only two years to live, I was very depressed, and sometimes music gave me some relief."

The club was too packed that night for me to use my wheelchair, so I left it in the trunk of the car and struggled in with my two canes. With a little luck, I wouldn't have too far to go. But the club was so crowded, there wasn't an empty seat in sight. I managed to lean against the bar, clutching my canes, looking for a chair. I pulled myself in as close as I could, afraid that someone in a hurry would accidentally knock me over.

Then I spotted a woman nearby who stood up as if getting ready to leave. I made my way in her direction. "Excuse me, ma'am. Do you need someone to keep that chair warm?"

She smiled and replied, "I was going to make that suggestion."

I gratefully plopped my numb body into the chair and breathed a sigh of relief. A few moments later the woman came back. She'd found another chair and was dragging it behind her. She sat down beside me and extended her hand.

"My name's Carolyn," she stated. "I'm so glad you're here. It was meant that we should be talking tonight. There are no accidents."

Meant to be talking? What was that supposed to mean? At some other time, I might have said something like, "Yeah, right," and rolled my eyes. But tonight I was grateful for the company.

Carolyn was kind, easy to talk to, and attractive—a good diversion from my troubling thoughts—and I began to feel very comfortable with her. She asked about my canes, and I found myself telling her about my MS and my frustrations and disappointments with conventional medicine. Finally I told her about my doctor's dismal prognosis for my future.

Carolyn listened compassionately. She told me she was a Doctor of Naturopathy, the equivalent of an MD in alternative medicine, and had a clinical practice in Australia. She talked a great deal about strengthening the immune system, and the need to treat the cause of an illness instead of just the symptoms. Even from my scientist's perspective, I could see some logic to that.

As the evening progressed I found myself taking this stranger very seriously. She appeared intelligent and sincere. Yet, in spite of my admiration for her, I still could not completely turn off my scientific mindset. I kept sparring with her, lightly jabbing at the things she told me about her practice.

Finally, Carolyn turned to me and remarked, "Gary, for just once in your life, can you allow yourself to imagine that there are things that happen in the world that you can't necessarily prove with science?"

"You don't know how hard that is for me," I protested.

"Let me put it this way," she continued. "As a physicist, you admire Albert Einstein, don't you?"

"Most certainly. He was gifted with a great mind."

"Well, it was Einstein who said, 'Imagination is more important than knowledge.' Do you see any truth to that?"

I laughed. "That may be the one thing he said that I don't agree with. Carolyn, my whole adult life has been spent pursuing scientific proof. Unsubstantiated concepts worry me."

Undaunted, she continued. "And what would happen if you let go of that position? I'm not saying that there isn't any proof of what I've been talking about. But what if there isn't? What would happen if you made room for the possibility that there are things that are true but which can't be proved?"

Unsure of where she was going with this, I asked, "We're talking about me personally, right? About my MS?"

"We sure are."

I thought for a moment. "In order to imagine that there is a cure for my MS outside of the science of modern medicine, I would have to lay aside everything that I've ever believed to be true, the very foundation of my life. Frankly, that scares me."

Carolyn sat back and looked at me intently. "And what are you protecting with those beliefs?"

The question made me feel anxious. "I don't know."

"Yes, you do. Just look at whatever comes into your mind."

The music in the jazz bar seemed to fade into the background. At first I couldn't bring anything into focus. Carolyn patiently waited. Then I realized that I knew what I was protecting.

"It's the reality of my illness. I've tried to ignore it, forget about it, escape it. But it won't go away. It's here to stay, and I have to deal with it, but I don't know how. It scares me that nothing the doctors have done seems to work. But I have to believe that there's an answer somewhere, an answer that science, so far, hasn't been able to produce. I know that I don't want to give up. I don't want to die."

I could feel the black despair that always lurked close to the surface. Carolyn sat still and waited as I regained my composure.

"I just have to believe that there is help for me, somewhere out there," I sighed. "Somewhere."

To my everlasting surprise, Carolyn gave me an enormous smile and beamed, "Oh, Gary, you're going to get well!"

I was astonished by what she said. But in that moment, I felt my first sense of real hope.

As we continued to talk, Carolyn confessed she had a strong feeling that an Aboriginal healer friend of hers might be able to help me. His name was Ray, and he spent part of the year living and working in an apartment in Brisbane, Australia, and the other part living with his tribe in the Outback. If I was willing to travel to Australia, he might be able to help me.

Carolyn could give me no guarantees that Ray could cure me, but that spark of hope I had felt continued to grow. Before we parted that night, I got Ray's telephone number in Australia; though, I imagined I would probably tear it up in the clear light of day.

The next day I pulled out the slip of paper and looked at it. This was insane. Forget Western medicine? Put my trust in some Aboriginal man in Australia, someone I'd never met? Pure idiocy. Then I dialed the number.

Ray was not home, so I left a message. The following day he had not returned my call, so I called again. This time he answered.

"I got your message," Ray stated. His voice seemed a bit rough and even annoyed. His accent was heavy, and I had to concentrate to understand him.

"Carolyn gave me your number," I explained.

"Oh yeah? How's she doing?" he responded curtly.

I described my situation and told him how I had come to meet Carolyn. I said that I hoped he'd be able to help me.

"Ahh . . . call me back in two weeks," he muttered abruptly.

"I don't have two weeks," I countered.

"What's so important?" he asked.

"My life."

There was a moment of silence.

"You've got time. Call me again in three days." Ray hung up.

I didn't know what to make of any of this and replayed the conversation over and over in my head. At least Ray had changed his mind, asking me to call him in three days instead of two weeks. This gave me hope. I couldn't wait for the days to pass.

On the third day I called as instructed. Ray seemed no friendlier than before.

"What makes you think we could help you?" he inquired.

I replied, "I'm only going on what Carolyn said."

"Well, maybe it's possible," he admitted. "There may be someone here who could help you. Call me again in three days." He hung up.

I felt unreasonably cheered. Ray had acknowledged that curing my

MS might be possible and that there might be someone who could help me in the Outback. It was a thin ray of hope, but it was a whole lot more than I was being offered by the medical community. I called Ray again three days later.

"When can you get here?" he demanded abruptly. Surprised at his sudden acceptance, I said, "Well, it will take me a few days to get a visa. I already have a passport. Then I'll have to get my airline tickets, so it'll probably be a week or two."

"You can do better than that. Call me when you're ready to go." He hung up.

The next day I took a two-hour trip to the Australian consulate in Los Angeles to acquire my visa. I used my frequent-flyer miles to get a roundtrip ticket with the return date open. I packed. In three days I called Ray and told him I was ready. This time he sounded a bit friendlier. He told me to call him when I arrived in Brisbane. He would take care of all my accommodations and ground transportation.

And that was it. I was headed for the Outback.

I was excited. My family and friends were appalled.

"Have you lost your senses?" my ex-wife asked. "How can you possibly make such a crazy decision based upon a chance meeting with some woman in a jazz lounge?" Thinking that it might dissuade me from going, she flatly refused to go with me.

I told her I would go alone.

"You're not in any shape to travel anywhere, let alone take an eighteen-hour flight all by yourself," she argued. "What if you get to Australia and are too ill to continue?"

"It's a risk I'll take," I insisted.

I told some of my closest friends what I was going to do, and they assumed I had gone off the deep end. "The medical treatment you receive here in the United States is the best the world has to offer," one of them contended. "You're chasing after a pipe dream. You're my friend, Gary, and I don't want to see you get hurt."

Ultimately there was no one who would go with me. Some claimed it was because of other commitments, but I think they all assumed I would give up the trip if I had to do it alone. It made me sad to realize that, all through my life, when push came to shove, I always seemed to be alone. I was certainly alone with my MS, and I was going to be alone on this trip to Australia.

But I was determined to go. Despite the apparent craziness of the situation, I knew there was something for me in the Outback. Just what it was, I didn't have a clue. But for once in my life, I wasn't being ruled by my mind. I was acting on something else, a gut feeling, a voice inside that told me to make this trip. There was no stopping me.

As I lay in bed the night before I was to leave, I thought of all that had happened in just over a week. I was a little apprehensive, but I was also excited. I felt that I had been given a huge gift. Carolyn's comment, "there are no accidents," suddenly took on new meaning. Perhaps there was a power at work that was more than I could know.

The next day I was wheeled aboard a plane headed for Australia. I was so weak by now that I was unable to use my canes to maneuver, and so my wheelchair was placed at the end of an empty row of seats in the back of the aircraft. That's where I'd spend the entire flight, sitting in my wheelchair without head or shoulder support.

The plane was full of people. Often in the past when traveling on business, I had deliberately avoided conversation with people seated next to me. Now I longed to feel less isolated. Looking up the long aisle of the airplane gave me the perfect vantage point for seeing all that went on, but left me with no way to be a part of anything.

After a fourteen-and-a-half-hour flight, I landed in Sydney at 10:30 p.m. local time. In three and a half hours, I boarded the connecting flight to Brisbane, and then I was there. Finally. And so tired I could hardly lift my hands.

An airline steward wheeled me off the plane, collected my luggage, assisted me through customs, and took me to a telephone. After I had made the call to Ray and gotten a reassuring message on his answering machine, the steward hung up the phone for me. He then picked up my suitcase and indicated he'd leave it at the taxi stand.

I watched him walk quickly away, too astonished to try to summon him back. By this time I was so tired, I could hardly force my numb arms to turn the wheels of my chair. I had never bought an electric chair because to me that represented the last defeat. Now I devoutly wished I could just push a button and propel myself toward the exit.

After forty minutes of struggle, I made it to the taxi stand. The men at the stand picked me up and wedged my 6' 2", 180-pound frame into the back of a station wagon, and drove me to my hotel. There the doorman and the taxi driver managed to get me back into my chair. I didn't have enough control over my hands to even sign my name to the hotel registry. All I could manage was the semblance of an *X*. When I got to my room, I fell onto the bed and went straight to sleep with my clothes on.

"I think you know the rest of the story," I told Rose. "Ray came by the next morning, loaded me and my stuff into his car, bounced me for seven hours over some of the worst roads I have ever seen, and delivered me to a room with the hardest bed I've ever slept on."

She laughed. "Did the hard bed keep you awake?" she asked.

"Actually, no," I answered. "I slept like a baby."

"So, Gary," Rose continued, "do you know why you trusted Carolyn and Ray enough to make this journey?"

I thought about it. "Not really," I replied. "There was something inside me that just responded. When Carolyn told me that I was going to get well, I believed her. I have no idea why. I just did."

I shook my head. "And Ray was a real bear when I first talked to him on the phone, but there was still something in me that trusted him. And when I finally met him in person, I felt like I'd known him all my life. It's unusual for me, because I'm normally a pretty reserved person."

Rose nodded. "Gary, you've certainly demonstrated a lot of willingness. But I want you to know that the most impressive willingness was not that you traveled thousands of miles, as hard as that was, but that you trusted a part of yourself that didn't deal in hard facts. You were willing to trust your intuition. You were willing to at least gamble that there were things beyond what you could know with your logical mind."

She smiled. "Now we'll see if you are equally as willing in other areas."

With that somewhat mysterious remark, Rose got up to leave. Just then, Ray came through the door to wheel me back down the path to my hut.

It was hard to believe the day had passed so quickly, but the sun was already sinking behind the distant scrub trees on the horizon. Back at my hut, Ray lit a candle. He brought a dinner of fruit and more grubs for both of us, then sat on the stump in the room as we silently ate.

He stretched, leaned back, and inquired, "Well, what did you learn today?"

"I learned about the first Essential of Healing—Willingness."

"So, are you willing to get well?"

"Well, I got here, didn't I?" I was feeling mildly annoyed at hearing this question for the second time. "Isn't that being willing?"

"You think that's all it takes, just getting here?" Ray made a dismissive gesture.

Now I was angry. How could he possibly know what I'd gone through to get here? My family had done everything they could to talk me out of going. My colleagues thought I was crazy. Not one person was willing to come with me. That plane trip, all alone, had been like a metaphor for my whole life.

"Do you know what it took me to get here?" I asked Ray.

"Not much. You used your frequent-flyer points. You had vacation time coming. So, where'd it cost you anything?"

"Do you know what it takes to get frequent-flyer points?" I questioned, steaming. Over the last five years, I'd flown all over the world to earn those points, supporting my numb legs with two canes when I could still stagger, and spending the rest of my time in a wheelchair, all in a desperate attempt to keep my business going.

"You sit on an airplane to get your points. I call those "butt" points. Let me tell you, Mate, that's not willingness."

At that point, I really wanted to tell Ray to fuck off. I was hot and tired, sticky with sweat in the stuffy little hut, and I just wanted some comfort or relief. I had looked forward to a relaxing evening of small talk with my new friend, not this pointless baiting. Ray couldn't possibly understand what I'd been through. He didn't really know me.

But he was my way in and way out of here, my only real ally besides Rose. I had to trust him. I bit my tongue and tried to swallow my anger. "So you tell me. What *is* willingness?"

Ray leaned forward and put his hand on my forearm. "For you, Gary, the question is, are you willing to feel? Are you willing to face your emotions? That's at the center of all of your problems."

When Ray asserted this, I wanted to argue, tell him he was wrong. But I couldn't. He had me pegged. The anger went out of me like air from a balloon.

I looked at him. "I'm willing," I affirmed, "but I don't know how. I'm willing to learn."

Ray studied me with his one good eye, then nodded. He inquired in a suddenly kind voice, "Want to tell me about your kids, Mate?" He urged me to talk about my two failed marriages and my strained relationship with my son and daughter.

As I talked I found that I was less analytical, less detached, and could begin to feel some of the pain that I carried around those issues. There was nothing dramatic. I didn't break into tears. But something was stirring. I had said I was willing to feel my emotions, and I was beginning to feel. But when we bid good night I was relieved to be alone. Alone and not being asked to deal with my emotions. Just alone with my thoughts.

As I prepared for bed, the little hut was stiflingly hot. The sun's descent had done little to cool the intense heat of the day, and there was no breeze. There was nothing to wash with, but I was too tired to care. Hygiene wasn't a big priority to me just then. Besides, there was no way I was going to get undressed, or even take off my shoes. I didn't want any large insects, which my numb feet wouldn't be able to feel, climbing into my shoes during the night.

I pulled my backpack off my wheelchair to use as a pillow and awkwardly lowered myself onto the board, jostling my catheter tubes down to the bottom of the pack. Then I lay still, listening to the sounds of the Outback. As the darkness settled, I began to hear the strange calls of nocturnal animals as they awakened and began to move about. I recognized none of them and lay there trying to calm myself into sleep.

Just then a hoarse, hacking roar shattered the night. I froze on my bed. The sound was like a cross between a grizzly bear and a jaguar. I knew that Australia had neither of those animals, but I couldn't imagine what could make such a terrifying sound. In a panic, I fumbled for my wheelchair and pushed it toward the open door of my hut to provide some protection.

I lay there listening to my heart pound, and then I heard the sound again, this time closer.

I was terrified. I tried to push the feeling away, to talk myself out of it, to deaden it. But it wouldn't go away. I could feel fear in every fiber of my being.

I closed my eyes and began to pray. "God, I'm all alone here, and my last hope for life is in this strange place. You brought me here for some purpose. Did I come this far just to be killed?"

And then, amazingly, I heard myself saying, "Well, if I'm supposed to die now, so be it."

As I decided that it was okay for me to die, the terror subsided and I began to feel a sense of peace. At that moment I knew, beyond all logic, beyond all knowing, that I was exactly where I needed to be. I had been driven by God and the events of my life right to this point. I was here for a specific reason, although I didn't know what that reason was. And I was willing to accept whatever it was that God had planned. I was willing to do whatever it took. And if that meant feeling all of my feelings, I was willing to do that.

I heard the roar again, and to my relief, this time it was farther away. I opened my eyes and turned my head toward the window. The stars, set against the blackness of the dimensionless backcountry sky, shone more vividly than I had ever seen them before. Time seemed to stand still. I felt strangely comforted and peacefully drifted off to sleep, waiting to see what God had in store for me.

4

AWARENESS

When I woke up the next morning, my wheelchair was across the room, blocking the doorway. I didn't know how I would get to it. I didn't want to call for help and embarrass myself, admitting how afraid I'd been of the monstrous roar in the night. And I wanted to rely on myself.

But no matter how I twisted myself on my bed, I could not get close enough to grab hold of the chair. I had no idea how long it would be before Ray showed up, and I desperately wanted off the hard sleeping platform before he arrived. It was clear that if I wanted to reach the chair, I was going to have to crawl to it.

I was determined to be sitting in that chair when Ray got here. So I struggled with my uncooperative, numb legs, finally pulling myself off the eighteen-inch platform. I landed hard on the dirt floor, scraping my back on the side of the bed in the process. Once down, I scooted on my butt, inch by inch, dragging and pushing the dead weight of my torso to the base of my wheelchair. Then I locked the brakes and began the process of pulling myself up into the seat. I tried and failed several times, sliding off the edge of the chair and landing with a heavy thud back onto the hard floor.

Fighting panic, I began to sweat in the morning heat. I really did not want Ray to find me in this situation. I didn't want him there watching me. Ray has a deliciously wicked sense of humor, and I did not want to be on the receiving end of it. And even if he offered to help, it would still be difficult for a man so much smaller than myself to lift me.

Finally, I managed to pull myself into the seat and began dusting myself off, trying to hide the evidence of my bad judgment from the night before. As soon as I got myself into some kind of presentable order, I spun the chair around to wheel myself outside. To my surprise, there, standing in the doorway, was a boy of about eleven or twelve. I felt a flash of embarrassment, sure that he had seen me crawling across the floor and struggling to get into the chair. Unsure of what to do, I simply said hello.

He bowed with a strangely reverent expression, and voiced something in his own language.

Before I could respond, the boy turned and disappeared.

"Morning, Mate!" It was Ray peering into the doorway now. Had he seen what just happened? He gave no indication, merely brought me my breakfast and wheeled me off to see Rose.

Another day baking in her little healing hut, only this morning I was Willing, and eager to tackle the second essential—Awareness.

Rose didn't seem surprised to hear about my conversation with Ray the night before, and the insights I'd gained about true willingness. I wasn't ready to share my fright about the wild animal, but managed to explain that I'd turned my fate over to God.

"That's wonderful, Gary," she responded. "Now you're ready for the next step to Awareness. The more aware you become, the faster your healing will take place, because awareness helps us see things differently.

"When you are aware of something, then you have less reason to fear it," Rose clarified, giving me a sideways look. "For most of us, life is like looking through a small hole in the wall at something beyond us. Everything outside of your limited scope of vision makes you feel uncomfortable because you're not familiar with it. It's a bit scary. Awareness helps you to expand your perception and release the fear."

I wasn't sure if she somehow knew about my panic in the night, but I wasn't about to bring it up. "So what do I need to become more aware of?" I asked instead.

"Well, for one thing, your relationship with your father."

It wasn't the answer I wanted to hear. I just wanted to forget about my father.

"There's still a lot of fear about your father that's lodged in your body," Rose advised. "Is there a specific incident that often comes up when you think of your father?"

I thought for a moment.

"Yes," I replied, somewhat bitterly, "the time he gave me the name 'birdbrain.'"

"Tell me about it."

Reluctantly, I complied. It was not a pleasant memory.

"It happened when I was about twelve years old," I told her.

My father had taken my younger brother and me with him to check on the tenants at my grandmother's property. I was sitting up front with my father, and my brother was in the back seat of our powder-blue 1955 Ford Galaxy 500, my father's pride and joy. As we pulled up to Grandma's house, we parked curbside behind a black panel truck. My father, who was already drunk, stumbled out of the car and ordered us to stay put.

As he began to walk up the pathway to the house, the driver of the parked truck, who apparently hadn't seen us pull up behind him, began to back up directly toward our car. I sat frozen in the front seat, waiting for the impending doom of the crash.

The next few moments happened quickly, but in my mind they seemed to occur in slow motion. My father turned upon hearing the sound of the starting engine and saw the moving truck and oblivious driver. Then he saw me, frozen in the front seat, and a look of rage came over his face. He dashed back, jerked open the car door, and jammed his hand down on the horn. The driver of the panel truck slammed on his brakes, just missing the front end of our Ford.

Now that disaster had been avoided, my father turned to me. I expected the worst and ducked my head protectively beneath my arms. Furious, he yelled, "What's the matter with you? Couldn't you see that car? Why didn't you just honk the horn? You're nothing but a fucking birdbrain!"

Ever since I was a child, my father had called me names like "stupid," but from then on "birdbrain" was his favorite. He taunted me with it constantly. Even though he's dead now, that word still haunts me. I have always felt that I had to prove that I was smart, that I was competent. In short, that I wasn't a *birdbrain*.

I looked at Rose as I finished. "Not a great memory to have of one's father, is it?"

"No, but it's perfect for our purposes," she told me. "It was an incident that held a lot of fear and pain for you as a child. In the next few days, I want you to continue to look at this incident and see if you can expand your awareness of it. See if you can look at it through a bigger hole in the wall."

I agreed, but I wasn't optimistic. I didn't see what more there was to be aware of, and I didn't like thinking about it.

By dinnertime that night, after more healing work with Rose including physical manipulations of my legs, I had pushed the memory of my father to the back of my mind. There was something more immediate in the forefront. The night before, I had heard that horrible roar and thought that I was about to end my days as a midnight snack for some wild animal. Obviously, I didn't. But I was facing another night with the creature somewhere outside my room, and no secure door, so I asked Ray about it.

"Uh, Ray, are there any dangerous animals out here?"

"What do you mean, Mate?"

"Well, last night I heard something, obviously big, making a lot of noise."

"Like what, Mate?"

I am not good at imitating animal noises, but after a few false starts, I managed to approximate a sound that was something like the beast that had frightened me.

"You mean, like this?" Ray asked, making a hoarse, hacking roar that was exactly like the creature.

"Yes, that's it!" I shuddered. "Should I be afraid? I mean, should I get a door put on my hut or something?"

"No, don't worry," Ray responded cheerfully. "This animal is so big, he wouldn't even bother with you."

His words gave me little comfort. I was about to protest again when he stood up and remarked he was going to get our dinner. I sat there alone, contemplating another night with that beast outside.

When Ray came back with our dinner bowls, he had a big brown bird on his shoulder.

"Who's your friend?" I asked.

"Oh," Ray replied, "you'll find out soon enough." He refused to say more, so we ate and talked about other things.

Then Ray noted, "I can see you're tired, Mate, so I'll say good night." He patted my back and left, still carrying the bird on his shoulder.

"I still don't know who your friend is," I called after him.

"You'll find out," he assured, and vanished into the dark.

I got myself ready for bed, lay down with my head on my pack, then closed my eyes and tried to relax into sleep. All of a sudden, right outside my window, I heard the terrible hoarse, hacking growl of the huge animal Ray had told me about. It was so close, I was sure it was going to come into my hut.

"Ray!" I shouted. "Ray! Somebody! Help me!"

Just then I heard Ray laughing his head off outside my window.

"What the fuck are you doing?" I yelled at him.

He came back in, shaking with laughter, the bird still sitting on his shoulder. "Meet my mate," he announced.

"You mean that *bird* is what is making that horrible sound?" I felt incredibly foolish, but weak with relief.

"Yep, that's the sound of the fierce kookaburra bird." Ray laughed. "He has a big bark, but no bite—just like some people."

He grinned at me and left, the bird sitting peacefully on his shoulder.

I relaxed on my bed, laughing. And then I thought of my father. And suddenly Rose's hole in the wall was bigger. Although my father had been a small man, only 5' 4" tall, he had kept the entire family terrorized. All of his sons were over 6 feet, but none of us had been able to stand up to him.

In a flash, I felt my lifelong terror of him begin to dissolve. My father's power had only been an illusion, and I could have walked away from it at any time. Now I saw what it had cost me to defend myself from him. The same walls that kept me safe from my father had kept me distant from everyone else—my wives, my children, my family, everyone.

I lay there and wondered whether I could begin to let down those walls. After all, there was nobody out there but a kookaburra bird.

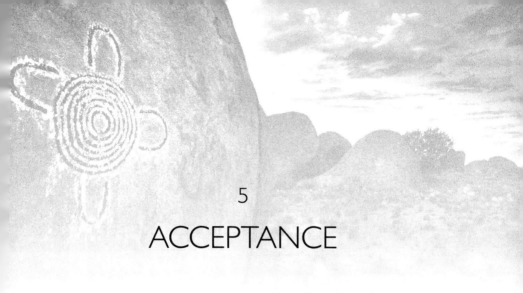

5

ACCEPTANCE

I woke up early the next morning and wheeled myself outside to enjoy the dawn light and the relative coolness before the day really heated up again. I nodded to a couple of women walking past my hut carrying the long woody straws I'd learned they use to draw up water from the underground stream that passes under the village. I nodded to the women, still not knowing a word of their language. They gave me smiles that managed to convey a great warmth and compassion without the need of words.

When I met Rose at her healing hut I told her that I had been given more insight into Willingness and Awareness by someone I'd met.

"And who was that?" she asked.

"A real birdbrain," I replied, grinning. "A kookaburra bird."

Rose laughed, the weathered creases around her eyes deepening, but somehow she looked younger. "I suppose Ray introduced you?"

I chuckled, then told her about my night of terror, and how I'd been willing to feel my fear rather than go numb when I heard the fierce "beast" outside. "When I allowed myself to experience it, I was able to let go of it, turn it all over to God, and sleep peacefully."

"That's a wonderful lesson in Willingness, Gary," she exclaimed. "And what was the lesson in Awareness?"

"When I learned that the 'beast' was a loudmouthed kookaburra bird, I could see my father through a larger peephole," I confided. "The man who was so terrifying in my childhood was just an insecure little bully."

Rose nodded. "Gary, those are great lessons. I think you're really clear about the first two essentials of Healing. Now you're ready for the next one. It's Acceptance. Gary, you need to accept yourself just the way you are, MS and all, before healing can happen."

She explained that Acceptance frees us to move on. She demonstrated this truth by writing something on a piece of paper, which she left lying on the table.

"Now," she pointed out, "if I write something on this piece of paper here, something intended for the garbage, I can't put it in the rubbish bin until I pick it up."

Then she picked up the paper and threw it away. "Only when we have accepted something are we able to toss it away," she clarified. "We all have things about ourselves that are not pleasant to look at. But if we don't look—and if we don't accept—we can't heal. Only through *total and unconditional* acceptance of the self can healing take place."

"I don't know if I can accept my MS," I told her. "Isn't that what I'm here for—to fight it, to make it go away?"

"No," she contended. "You're here to accept it—and then let it go away. Acceptance is a hard lesson. But I think you've become more accepting of yourself, of your illness, in the short time that you've been here."

I thought about it. "You know, I think you're right. Actually, I was taught a lesson in acceptance by that same birdbrain."

Rose chuckled. "We're going to have to put that kookaburra bird on staff. How did he teach you about acceptance?"

"Well," I told her, "I'm embarrassed to admit it now, but when I heard that roar outside my window, I pushed my wheelchair across the room to block the door."

"Did you think that would stop the beast?" She grinned.

"I thought it might slow him down," I reasoned, laughing at the memory. Somehow this morning I wasn't ashamed to tell her about my ridiculous pride and the struggle with the wheelchair. And about that young boy who'd watched me with such a strangely reverent look.

"I cannot shake the image of that boy watching me. There was no judgment in his eyes. Just a calm acceptance." I closed my eyes and took a deep breath. "I've felt a lot of things from people when they see my condition. Usually it's pity. But there was none of that with this boy. No pity. No judgment. No nothing—just acceptance."

Rose gave me a gentle smile. "Sometimes our children are closest to the truth," she noted. "Perhaps seeing the acceptance in his eyes will help you learn to accept your MS—to actually pick it up so that you can eventually throw it away."

We worked more on Acceptance that morning. After we had taken a break for lunch, this time a piece of fruit and some unidentified insects, which I crunched down cheerfully, Rose asked me if I wanted to rest.

"No," I said. "If you feel like continuing, so do I." Then I added, with a touch of sarcasm, "Sitting in this wheelchair all day doesn't exactly tire me out."

She responded to the sarcasm immediately. "Gary," she replied, "one of the most important things that you can learn while you are here is that undesirable circumstances come into our lives not merely to make our lives difficult, but to teach us. I know that having MS is not pleasant for you, but if you can recognize that this is your ultimate learning lesson—given to you so that you can change, grow, and develop, both physically and spiritually—it will make your condition much easier to accept."

"I know you're right," I conceded, embarrassed. "I guess I just have trouble seeing what the lesson is."

"Then let's look at that." She studied me, neither smiling nor frowning, but somehow her penetrating gaze felt comfortable to me now.

"What *has* it taught you, Gary? Having MS?"

I sat quietly for a moment and thought about that. In my life before the MS struck, I had been intensely driven by my business, which designed microwave components for government defense projects. Most of the people I came into contact with were prospective business partners or clients, and I had seldom thought about the humanity of people. There wasn't much room for humanity in a roomful of people who, directly or indirectly, were dispassionately planning the potential deaths of millions.

"Well," I heard myself saying in a quiet voice, "I've learned a lot about compassion."

"Yes, that's right."

"If I didn't have MS, I would never have slowed down enough to really look at other people and their problems or feel a sense of empathy for their pain."

"That's right," agreed Rose. "And that's a very important lesson. You will make progress in accepting your MS if you can remember that we come into this life to learn lessons—lessons that will help us develop as human beings, lessons that will enable us to help others.

"What you are supposed to learn from your childhood and your MS and all of your life's experiences has to do with the pursuit of your gift. The growth you are accomplishing now is the key to its arrival."

"Gift? Pursuit of what gift?" I had no idea what she was talking about. I was in pursuit of health. That was it.

But Rose just smiled and said that I would understand more, later. She went on, "There are no such things as problems, Gary. Only chances to learn."

"So how do I get better at Acceptance?" I asked. "It doesn't come easy to me."

"Acknowledgment is one key," she explained. "Begin by acknowledging *everything* you've ever done. When you do this, it's an opportunity for you to feel pride in, and appreciate, your accomplishments. You can even make a list of them. When you learn how to acknowledge what you've done, you don't have to seek approval from anyone else, because you've learned how to give yourself praise and encouragement."

She told me that I could start by acknowledging myself for being in Australia and doing something about getting myself well.

"There are a lot of people sitting around in wheelchairs feeling sorry for themselves, but you are doing something about your illness," she told me. "We need to learn to praise ourselves for every single thing we do. The best method of disciplining children, or encouraging others, is to catch them doing something right and then praise them for it. So, catch yourself doing things right, and give yourself praise. Use this as a tool to help you focus on what's working in your life, rather than what's not working."

Then Rose told me to acknowledge all the people in my life who were helping or assisting me in some way—and that included negative people.

"If you have people in your life who are giving you a really hard time, acknowledge that they can teach you something," she advised. "Ask yourself what you can learn from them. It's better than wasting your energy saying, 'So-and-so is a real pain in the ass.' Sometimes people teach you things by being the opposite of what you want in your life, by being full of fear and hate. Negative as those people may seem, they help you by clearly showing you what you don't want to become."

"So I can acknowledge people for being negative role models?" I asked.

"Yes, but keep it to yourself." She smiled.

Another way to increase Acceptance, she told me, was to practice gratitude. "There are two parts to this. First, give thanks for all the good that you have in your life right now.

"Second, when you look at the parts of your life that seem to be negative, understand that they have the potential to be transformed into incredible positive energy."

"So I should be grateful for the good and the bad?"

"Yes," Rose responded. "If you feel gratitude for everything you have, you will live your life in a state of continual affirmation."

"So how can I begin to be more grateful for MS?"

"You can begin by being grateful to your body, regardless of what is happening in it. Let's say you're having problems with your legs at the moment. Take the time to notice how you feel. Then you thank your body for hurting.

"When you have problems in your body, it's actually your body sending you a message to change your actions. If your best friend was giving you some good advice, wouldn't you thank him? Your body is also your best friend. Thanking it for sending you a message causes you to experience a change of consciousness in your entire body."

Rose told me to take a moment and notice the signals my body was sending me. Then she said, "Now close your eyes and say 'Thank you.' See how you change completely?"

As directed, I focused on the discomfort I was feeling in my legs and thanked my body. Surprisingly, I felt better, much calmer. "It's actually very restful and relaxing," I told Rose.

"Yes, it's a real relief. The more you show gratitude, the more good things you get back. Your cells are able to pick up new positive beliefs and positive energy, making you a whole being. So continue to notice and say thank you.

"If you have a pain somewhere, notice how it feels, and then thank your body. Take a deep breath, and let it out. Then notice and thank again. Keep doing that until the pain subsides, until you feel really good."

Even though I had been breathing and offering gratitude during the whole time Rose was talking, there was still a persistent dull throb in my left leg that wouldn't stop. "But what if the pain doesn't go away?" I questioned. "My leg still hurts. Maybe I'm not doing this right."

"If the pain persists, you then ask yourself, 'What do I need to do? Legs, what do I need to do to support you in that chair?' It's as if you are asking your illness for an answer. You may not get the answer straight away, but it will come eventually. That's how Einstein got some of his best ideas. He'd just ask, and eventually the answer would come to him. It doesn't matter what we call the energy force that delivers the message, the important thing is that we listen to it."

A final key to Acceptance, Rose told me, was patience. She inquired, "Gary, do you know what the term 'lag' means?"

"To be lagging behind something?"

"Yes, that's right, but I'm using it in a slightly different sense. In your case, 'lag' means the distance between the first point and the second point, where you're headed for now and where you've been. 'Lag' represents whatever you want to achieve.

"But this is where patience comes in. You don't know how long it is going to take for you to reach your goal. You have to have patience with yourself because you can't achieve your objective straight away. The results you want may take some time."

That evening, I sat and talked with Ray about the lessons of the day. I almost told him about my experience of crawling for the chair that morning, but I thought better of it.

As we sat in the open hut enjoying the somewhat cooler air of the evening, two tribesmen came to the door. They were both very dark, wearing nothing but loincloths, their splayed, callused feet covered with the red dust of the Outback. To my surprise, they both began bowing to me. One uttered something in the "pidgin" English that I couldn't understand. The men bowed again and left.

I was taken aback. "What's going on?" I asked Ray. "Why did they bow? What did he say?"

"He said they have come to honor you."

To honor me? That seemed like a strange thing to say.

"What is there to honor about this broken man? I'm the one who is honored. I never imagined I'd get a chance to be in such a place, let alone have a healer giving me her undivided attention for ten hours a day."

"They honor the presence of the Big Guy, of the God that is in you," Ray murmured quietly. "They know that you are here because it is His will. We have known for quite a while that you would come."

I remembered Rose's comment from a few days ago: "We've been expecting you for months."

"I'm having trouble understanding what you mean by that," I confessed. "I didn't know that I was coming here months ago. How could you and everyone in this village have known this before I did?"

"We were told you would come. Gary, everything that happens in this universe is connected in ways you could never even imagine. All I can tell you at this time is that you are here for a purpose above and beyond your own healing. You were born with a gift, and you have come here so we can help you fulfill your destiny." Ray was very serious, looking intently into my eyes as he spoke.

Gift. There was that word again.

"What kind of gift could someone like me have to offer?" I asked, disbelieving. All my life, I had only seemed to make the people who became close to me sad, frustrated, or angry—my ex-wives, my kids, my mother, my siblings.

"We all have gifts, Gary," Ray replied with unusual gentleness. "God does not make empty vessels. We all have a destiny to fulfill, and the universe supports us in our journey. The gift you have been given is a healing gift."

Now I was positive Ray was mistaken. "Yeah?" I retorted bitterly. "Well, if I possess some kind of healing gift, then why can't I heal myself? Why am I so sick?"

Ray leaned in close to make his point. Staring me straight in the eyes, he explained, "Because the Big Guy needs you to understand that you must learn how to crawl, really crawl, before you can learn how to walk."

The power of his words struck me with such an impact that I couldn't even react. At the same time I was sure that somehow, some way, Ray *knew* about my crawling incident that morning.

Shortly after, Ray said good night, leaving me to prepare for bed and contemplate the events of the day. My thoughts were swirling in my head. I saw that Acceptance would be one of the hardest lessons to learn—but one of the most rewarding, if I could pull it off.

Could I accept that my illness had taught me valuable lessons? Could I be grateful for everything that came my way? Could I listen to my body and accept what it was telling me? And could I have patience? Could I accept that healing wouldn't necessarily happen according to a timetable I had chosen?

It was a daunting task. I didn't know if I could do it. All I knew was at that moment I was very grateful to be where I was, learning what I was learning. Maybe, emotionally, I was barely crawling. But that was how you learned to walk. And that was enough for now.

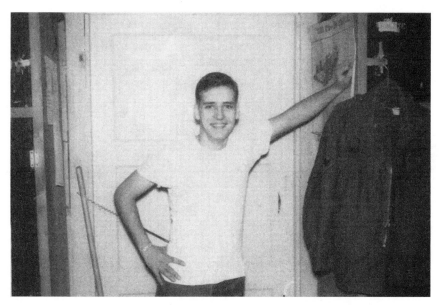

Young Gary Holz in the Army in the 1960s.

Gary Holz (right) as a young adult with now deceased brother Joe Holz (left).

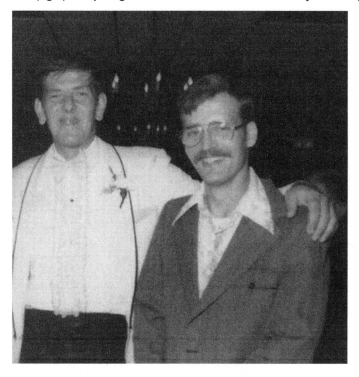

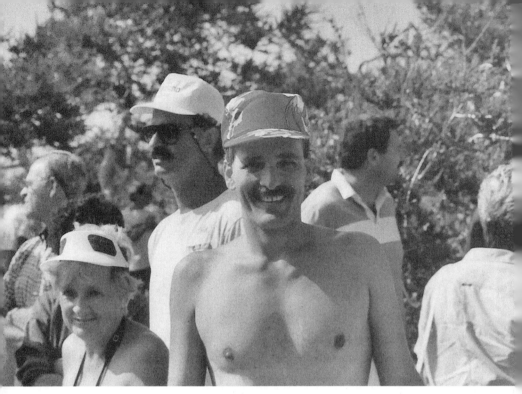

Gary Holz after completing the 26-mile open water Catalina Channel Marathon a few years prior to his diagnosis of MS.

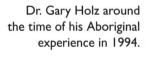Dr. Gary Holz around the time of his Aboriginal experience in 1994.

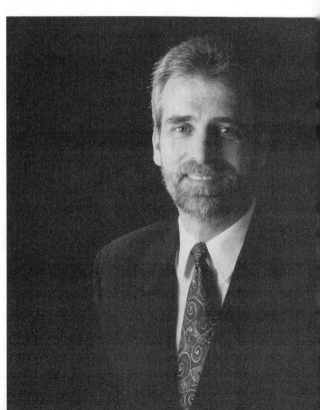

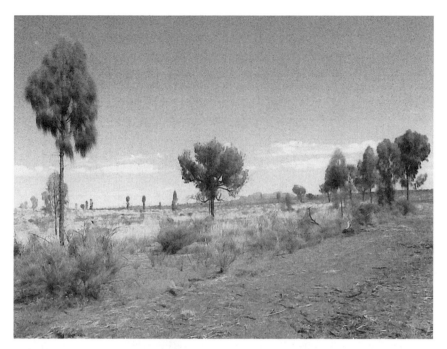

Outback desert, similar to the setting of Gary Holz's Aboriginal experience.
Photo by Robbie Holz.

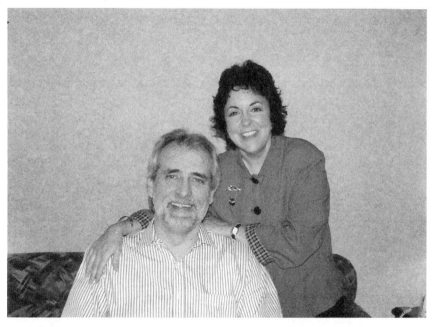

Several years after his Aboriginal experience, Gary Holz healed and happily
married to coauthor Robbie Holz.

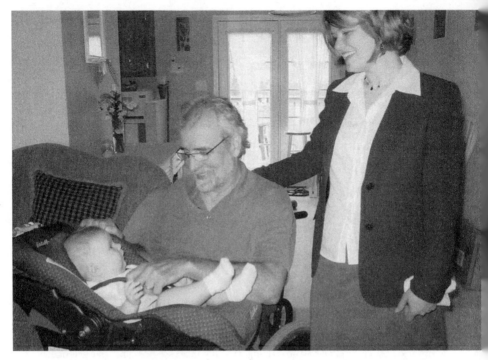

Gary Holz with his daughter Sonia Holz-Smith and his grandson Cooper Smith. (After his Outback experience, Gary healed his relationship with his estranged daughter Sonia and met his grandson Cooper in 2005—living well beyond the doctors' 1994 prognosis of two years.)

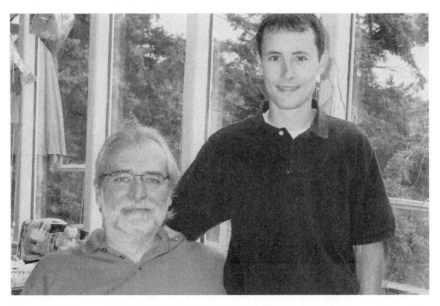

Gary with his son Chris Holz in 2006. (After his Outback experience, Gary also healed his relationship with his estranged son Chris.)

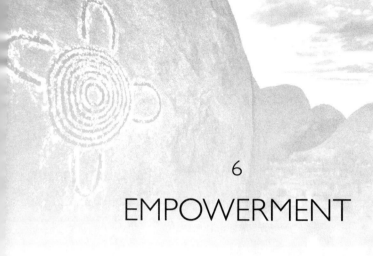

6

EMPOWERMENT

The next day a few men who'd been off on a hunting trip returned with some birds they'd caught. This seemed to be the occasion for another evening celebration. As I was feeling more comfortable with the people now, I rolled my chair over to join a group preparing for the gathering.

This time they were mixing some whitish clay with water to make a muddy sort of paint. Some of the children and men were painting each other's bodies in elaborate designs of lines, dots, and stars.

"Ray." I waved him over as I saw him passing. "What do the designs mean?"

Ray looked up and over to the side, addressing the air, "All these questions he's always asking! What are we going to do with him?"

I'd gotten used to his little conversations with himself, so ignored this remark. "Really, Ray. Can you ask them for me?"

He shook his head. "No need, Gary. It's just like the songs and dances they'll be doing tonight. It's all gratitude. They're thanking the Big Guy for giving us life, giving us everything we need." He made an expansive gesture that included the poor huts of the village and the bare stretch of the Outback with its red dirt and scraggly brush.

I felt humbled with the realization of what these people regarded as wealth—pretty sparse to my Western thinking. Yet, I was starting to see just how much they did have cause to celebrate.

A little girl ran over to watch the body painting, leaning against my wheelchair and giving me the open look of curiosity I was getting used to.

She muttered something to one of the painters, and he reached up to dab a spot of white over her heart.

I suddenly noticed how beautiful she was, with her dark skin and big gleaming eyes.

She spun around to look at me as I thought that, and her face broke into the biggest grin I'd ever seen. She laughed in delight, jumping up and down. She shyly squeezed my finger, and then ran off giggling.

"She says, 'Thank you,'" Ray told me.

By now I had made some progress in understanding the first three Essentials of Healing—Willingness, Awareness, and Acceptance. I was ready for Empowerment, the one that Rose indicated was the most challenging.

"Empowerment is about taking back your power and taking responsibility for yourself," Rose explained in our next session. "You don't really have a word that translates this concept very well. Empowerment usually means giving power to someone else. There is no word that means reclaiming the power that is really yours. The closest one is 'taking responsibility,' but that expression is associated with duty and obligation. So we're going to use Empowerment, because the essence of this concept is power."

When we blame others for the conditions of our lives, Rose clarified, we are giving our power away. And when we give our power away, we're giving our energy away.

"No one can steal your energy," she remarked. "You must allow it to be taken. It is very important to know that no one can do anything to you unless you give him or her permission. And there are some things that many people do constantly that give away their power."

To demonstrate this, Rose asked me if I had ever had muscle testing done. I told her that I had not.

"Okay," she began. "Just hold your arm straight out from your body while I push down on it. This is not a test of brute strength; it's a test of energy. I will make a statement and when I say 'hold,' I want you to do your best to lock your arm at the shoulder. If this is a true statement, then your arm will stay locked in position. If the statement is false, your arm will automatically fall when I push down on it, even if I only touch it with one finger.

"We are not talking to your conscious mind now," Rose continued, "but to your subconscious mind, communicating through the agency of your body, which does not lie. I can ask you any question, and your body will tell me everything that I need to know."

I extended my arm and held hard while Rose pushed down. "That's it," she encouraged. "Don't forget to keep breathing, because if you're holding your breath, you are using brute strength against me. Okay, I want you to say: *My name is Gary.*"

As I said, "My name is Gary," she pushed down on my arm and it held firm.

"See? When you say that, your arm is strong because that's your name. Now say: *My name is Bill.* And hold."

"My name is Bill," I stated. To my surprise, hard as I tried, I couldn't hold my arm up.

"Your arm is giving way because you know this isn't your name."

We tried this technique with several other true and false statements, and the results were always the same. I started to laugh.

"I love how this works," I exclaimed.

"Now I am going to ask you a couple of questions to show you how we use our words to give away our energy," Rose informed. "I want you to say: *I apologize.* And hold."

"I apologize," I repeated, holding my arm out straight from my body.

Rose attempted to push it down, but it wouldn't budge. "See, that arm is holding nice and strong. Now I want you to say: *I'm sorry.*"

"I'm sorry," I repeated.

This time she was able to easily push down my arm. "Do you see how your arm is giving way? This is what happens when you say *I'm sorry.* You are giving away your power. Never say *I'm sorry.* Always say *I apologize.*"

She directed me to position my arm again. "Now I want you to say: *I'm doing my best.* And hold."

"I am doing my best," I repeated, and my arm held firm.

"A strong response again," Rose observed. "Now I want you to say *I'm trying.*"

"I'm trying," I stated, as she pushed my arm down easily.

"Your arm is giving way again," Rose noted. "That's what happens when you are *trying.* Always say *I am doing my best.*

"If you apologize and are doing your best, you are giving good, positive, strong responses. People say *I'm sorry* and *I'm trying* all the time, but these phrases are full of negative energy because they show weakness. You send the message that you're sorry for existing. You are therefore giving away your power. It is important to remember that your words and your thoughts contain your energy. Do not be careless with them. Use them for positive purposes."

As I reflected on what Rose was saying, I realized the truth of it. My whole body felt different when I said *I'll do my best* as opposed to *I'll try.* If such a simple change in vocabulary could make such a difference, I was eager to hear more.

Rose told me that one way to understand responsibility is to see that there are basically three types of people in the world.

"The first type is the Victim," she explained. "These are the kinds of people who say, *Poor me. I feel so sorry for myself. Please help me. Rescue me. Do things for me.*"

I had to laugh at how comical she sounded mimicking these pitiful voices.

"Rescuers are the second type of people," Rose continued. "They rescue the Victims! The reason people rescue is threefold. First, they want approval. Second, they want praise—pats on the back. Those two reasons make them feel good and important."

"But the third reason people become Rescuers is that when you rescue others, you are in control of them. Sometimes this control is obvious, and other times it's very subtle."

"But is it always bad to be a Rescuer?" I asked. "If it makes people feel good and useful, and helps some people, what's so terrible about it?"

"The problem, Gary," she told me, "is that Rescuers soon assume the role of the people they are helping. Do you think the victims are grateful for their interference? No! The Rescuers get kicked in the gut because, sooner or later, the Victims begin picking up on the fact they are being controlled and back off.

"The Rescuer, who has been such a nice guy and was doing such nice things for the Victim, is now hurt that the Victim doesn't want to be rescued anymore. In a sense, he becomes a Victim."

Rose related the third type of person is the Master, the kind of person who is master over himself, master of his destiny. "The Master is the guy who makes things happen."

"So how do I become a Master?"

"By being neither a Victim nor a Rescuer," she answered. "You have to be vigilant at first. After a while it becomes part of your world view. If you go back to your old patterns of negative thinking, or if you make a mistake, don't give yourself a hard time about it. Acknowledge it and move on. If you are aware of it, you can change it."

Rose added that the more I practiced this technique, the more I would be thinking and believing in a positive mode. Being positive didn't mean evading the truth. "The most important thing you can do, Gary, is to always be honest and true to yourself. Don't ever lie to yourself. Don't pretend that your disease isn't happening or that your life is really okay. That's a form of nonacceptance."

"I'm very good at denial," I admitted. "Four months into my second marriage, my wife and I knew we weren't going to make it, but I just let it drag on instead of doing anything about it. Even after we went into counseling, I kept telling myself that everything would be all right if only *she* would change.

"Then when I first began experiencing episodes of MS, even though two doctors at two different hospitals told me my diagnosis, I still didn't want to believe it. I kept telling myself it was only a pinched nerve."

Rose nodded. "Many people practice denial. It's a basic human survival mechanism. Usually we deny something because it's too painful to look at.

"You're the type of person who is afraid to get too much into your feelings. When you do get emotional sometimes, you think, 'Oh God, this hurts. I wish I was back in blissful ignorance.' The correct response to that is, 'No way! There's no way I want to go back to being ignorant ever again.' And then, once you get through the negative emotions—acknowledging them, processing them, digesting them—you will feel better, lighter."

After this session with Rose, I spent a lot of time thinking about the issue of Empowerment—taking personal responsibility for my life—and how to be a Master, not a Victim or Rescuer. The primitive conditions at the village gave me plenty of opportunities to put this concept into practice.

As the sweltering heat seemed to increase daily in intensity, the limitations of my physical body continued to plague me. The heat left my muscles limp, making it difficult for me to have any sense of control. The lack of sensation in all parts of my body made every movement an effort. Although the work that Ray and Rose were doing with me required almost no physical exertion, the emotional, spiritual, and conceptual changes I was going through were leaving me exhausted at the end of each day.

I hadn't had a bath in days, and I knew I was beginning to smell badly. My shoes sitting on the footrests of my wheelchair were covered with red dirt and dust, even though I had not set foot upon the ground.

It certainly was a temptation to think *poor me,* but as soon as the thought came to my mind, I could hear Rose's voice mimicking the pitiful sounds of the Victim: "*Poor me. I feel so sorry for myself. Please help me. Rescue me. Do things for me.*"

Ray had shown me where I could clean myself with a makeshift shower, which consisted of a tarp that held water. Once you were underneath it, you could pull a cord and allow the water to flow over you for a moment. But I would have to undress outdoors in plain sight of everyone, and then sit under the tarp to soap up and rinse.

Even though I knew I desperately needed a shower, my fear of being naked in front of the villagers—of making a spectacle of myself as I tried to either drag or wheel myself into the shower, and then struggle back into my clothes in plain sight of all—had overridden my desire for cleanliness.

So what should I do? I didn't want to be a Victim. I didn't want to be rescued. But I wanted a bath. How would a Master handle the situation? I wasn't sure, but I decided to simply tell the truth and ask for what I needed.

"Uh, Ray," I began that evening, "maybe you've noticed that I haven't been using the shower."

Ray nodded. "I was wondering about that, Mate."

"Well, it's because I'm too embarrassed to take off my clothes in front of everybody and roll myself in there. Could I ask you a big favor? Could you bring me a bucket of water and a washcloth so that I can bathe in here?"

Ray looked at me kindly. "That's a big step for you, Gary. Admitting to your vulnerability and asking for help. I'll be right back."

In a few moments, Ray returned with not one, but two buckets of water, a couple of clean rags, and a small bar of soap, all of which he carefully placed on the tree trunk designated as my table. "Here you go, Mate. One for washing and one for rinsing. If there's nothing else I can get for you, I'll see you in the morning."

"Thanks," I sighed from the bottom of my heart.

I waited until it was completely dark and the village had quieted down for the night. Then, by moonlight, I prepared for the first bath I had taken in days. I can't even begin to describe what it felt like to be able to strip in the privacy of my hut, soap up my stinking, sweat-soaked body, rinse, and get clean again. I felt deliciously cool, in spite of the heat—like someone who had been reborn.

I finally took off my shoes after days of wearing them and ended my sponge bath by soaking my hot, gritty feet in the remainder of the water. I thought about putting my shoes back on again, but decided that I'd let them air for a week or so. That night I lay down to the most blissful and refreshing sleep I'd had in a long, long time.

The next day, Ray arrived with a breakfast of quail eggs. He glanced down at my glaringly white feet and then back up at my smiling face. "Just wondering, Mate, when was the last time those feet saw the light of day?"

"You're not going to get to me this morning, Ray," I vowed, laughing. "I feel much too good to allow that. Besides, we both know now that I've learned to crawl and that I'm preparing to walk. And when I do, I want to feel the dirt of Australia between my toes."

I tried wiggling my toes to show their agreement, though I did not get much of a response. But Ray laughed with me and proclaimed, "It's going to happen, Mate. It's going to happen."

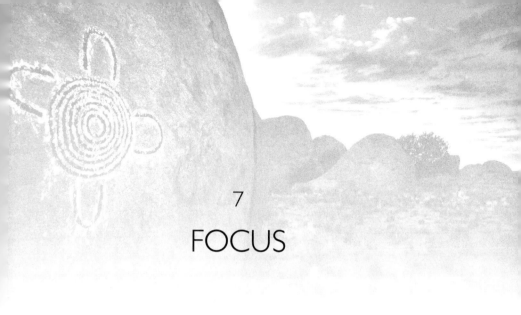

7

FOCUS

One day began to melt into the next as I settled into "Aboriginal time." It didn't seem important to keep track of the date, as I studied and began to live in the present, not rushing forward as I'd always done.

Those days in the Outback began to fall into a routine. After working with Rose for eight to ten hours, a combination of the spiritual lessons and physical exercises for my legs, if I wasn't too tired I'd have a bedtime discussion with Ray about what I was learning. As I lost my shyness around the other villagers, I began wheeling myself to the central gathering place of the compound to share the evening meal with them.

Ray would bring me a wooden bowl filled with meat or grubs and maybe a fruit or vegetable, which we ate with our fingers, most often in silence. That silence was beginning to "sound" fuller to me, as I sensed the unspoken communication and unity of the villagers. Once in a while someone said something aloud and Ray would translate for me. It was frequently a statement telling me how welcome I was among them, and I always nodded in grateful acknowledgement.

One morning Rose began by telling me that we would cover the last of the Five Essentials of Healing in our session. Then we would have the groundwork in place for the deeper healing to begin.

I was excited and somewhat confident, since I knew that the last

Essential was Focus. If there was anything I was good at, it was being able to focus. What I found, to my surprise, was that I could focus obsessively on some things, but I had very little ability to focus on what would heal me.

To begin our session, Rose told me a story about her nephew Luke. "He's only sixteen years old," she explained, "but he's been a champion canoeist for many years. Recently, I watched him race a marathon down the Gold Coast. It was very interesting. He took off from the starting point, paddled all day, got some sleep, and then paddled again all the next day. He's doing this, mind you, in the K1, a really unstable canoe that not too many people use.

"When he completed the race, he came in almost five minutes ahead of the closest competitor. And this is a kid who has been trained by a rookie coach competing against canoeists who have been trained by Olympic athletes. I ran over to give him a big hug, and I asked, 'Luke, what's it feel like to be the champion? What does it feel like to be the best in Australia?'

"He usually doesn't say much, and this time was no different. He looked at me, smiled, and replied, 'Normal.'

"It struck me that this is the true power of knowing. My nephew knows he's a champ, he knows he's a winner. It's all a matter of focus. There is a law of attraction at work. Very simply, it is whatever you focus on, you will attract."

This was a very different slant on focusing, and one that I was not very comfortable with. If I looked at what I had attracted in my life—MS, failed marriages, alienated children—I must not have been focusing on the right things. But I was certainly interested in attracting something different, so I listened intently.

"Always focus on wellness as opposed to illness," Rose told me. "Look at the problem, accept it, but don't dwell on it. Focus on the healing. Focusing on healing has to do with placing your attention on *what you want* as opposed to *what you don't want*. You have a situation or condition in your life or in your body, like your MS, that you want to change, and you decide that you're really Willing. You become Aware of the condition, you Accept it, and you take Responsibility for it. When you've looked at the problem this way, you can begin to *Focus* on what your solution might be.

"It's not a matter of learning how to focus," she added. "It's a matter of controlling what we focus on. There is a very human tendency to focus on the negative—the fight we just had, the job we don't like, some terrible situation in our life, a new wrinkle or gray hair.

"Have you ever tried to quit thinking about some problem? For most people, it's impossible. Their minds keep returning, replaying the tape. We focus to the point of obsessing. And the more we focus on the negative, the more we attract it. The key is learning how to control what we focus on and to focus on what we want in life, not what we don't want. In other words, we need to be conscious about what we focus our minds on."

Rose explained that it was important not to use words like *wish* and *want* when focusing on our desired goal. "When you want to change something in your life, you don't *wish* and you don't *want*," she clarified. "Because if you do those things, nothing is going to happen. For example, I need $2.00 to purchase a new pen that I saw in a shop, but I don't have $2.00 at the moment. Now, if I say, *I wish I had that pen,* or *I want that pen, but I can't afford it,* what I'm doing is sending out the energy of lacking. I'm focusing on the lack of the pen, and that's what will usually come back—the lack of the pen."

"But if I say, *that pen is already mine, it's in the shop waiting for me, but I'm not in a position to have it yet,* the effect is more positive. The word *yet* is a very powerful word to add onto expressions of desire. If you say *I can't afford that,* you've closed the door on ever having it. But if you say, *I don't have it yet, but I will have it tomorrow when I have my $2.00,* then you leave the door open to possessing it when the conditions are right."

An important ingredient in setting a goal is setting a time frame for achieving it, Rose told me. "When people set goals, they often don't put deadlines on achieving those goals," she pointed out. "When we keep pushing our goals into the future, all we have accomplished is to postpone them. We have to focus not just on having the goal but on having it at some definite time."

She emphasized it was very important to understand that the human subconscious doesn't know the difference between something that's real and something that's envisioned or imagined. "If you say, *I have it now,* then the subconscious will *think* that you have it now," she stated. "You create the conditions for you to get what you want when you put out energy that says *it's already mine.* Then the universe, feeding on this energy, creates the conditions for you to have what you want in reality. So, never have a *want* or a *wish.* You fake it until you make it."

"Okay," I hesitated. "How's this? I already know I'm going to get well."

"Good," concurred Rose. "That's the right attitude. Now, do you remember the old joke about how many psychologists it takes to change a lightbulb?"

"Yes," I smiled. "It only takes one, but that's only if the lightbulb really wants to change."

"Right," laughed Rose. "And we're like lightbulbs, Gary. There may be one person who's stuck in the socket and doesn't want to change. He's lost all his energy and is useless to himself and everybody else. But there's another lightbulb that does want to change.

"Human beings, as a rule, don't want to change," she continued. "We dig in our heels and resist. Fear of change is the greatest disease of all, and the hardest to cure. It's not change itself that causes stress, it's our resistance to change. In order to begin healing we need to let go, stop fighting, stop resisting, accept what's happening, and then do something about it."

"I know that I want to change," I admitted.

"I know that, too, Gary," Rose affirmed. "That's all anyone can ask for. And you've got more help than you can possibly imagine."

"What do you mean by that?" I inquired. "What help are you talking about?"

"Gary, all healing really comes from God and from our connection with God," Rose answered. "We have all the answers we need inside of us to heal. We only have to learn how to access those answers. The secret is that you don't have to rely on just yourself, your own mind, and your experiences. All the intelligence in the entire universe is within you, Gary. You just don't know how to access it yet.

"Ultimately, we heal ourselves. Sometimes we are assisted by healers, but we don't always have to go to the doctor, the acupuncturist, or the physical therapist to be healed. We heal ourselves, and we can learn to do this more consciously. If we want to be healthy on every level, we need to learn to focus—to cultivate conscious awareness."

"So how do I do it? How do I tap into this intelligence that you say is within me?"

"Whether you've been aware of it or not, you have always been tapping into it for answers, at one time or another," Rose advised. "Did you ever get a sudden answer out of nowhere for a question you'd been puzzling over?"

"Yes, many times," I nodded. "Sometimes a client would come to me with a problem, and I'd see the solution before they even got done explaining what they needed."

"Exactly. It works the same way with your health. It's all a matter of becoming quiet enough to hear that voice within and then trusting it," Rose asserted. "You'll be able to do this easily before you leave. And you'll be able to use it to help others."

"Okay." I was skeptical, but willing to see how it all unfolded. "So is that all there is to it? Learning to listen to that little voice? And trust it?"

"Well, that's the first part. The next thing you need to do is to learn how to control your thoughts and expectations of what your reality will be. Our thoughts, beliefs, emotions, and words create our reality. So, if you can believe you've *created* your MS, then you can also start believing that you can *uncreate* it.

"That's a hard idea for most people to comprehend," Rose continued. "It's the law of attraction: You get back what you put out. Whatever we focus our attention on or put our energy into is what we automatically create. And the most powerful energies we should focus our attention on are love and forgiveness, of both ourselves and others."

"I'm sorry, but this sounds too simple," I protested. "There are a lot of self-help books in America that talk about the power of affirmations, and I've even tried reading a couple of them since I got sick, but they never seemed to work for me. Am I missing something here?"

"That's an honest question," Rose acknowledged. "And you're right. No one can change his basic programming through merely repeating positive affirmations. You must really believe, with your whole soul, the messages behind the affirmations, and live those messages in your daily life, for the reprogramming to be legitimate.

"However, even repeating the positive affirmation without entirely believing the message behind it is better than nothing. Doing that puts out positive energy, but that is only a stopgap measure. A more radical change in attitude is needed. Look at how many people in the world have good intentions, but can't seem to stop repeating the same patterns."

"I'm not really sure that I can do everything that you're saying," I confessed, "but if you're willing to help me, I'm willing to try." Then I caught myself. "Let me rephrase that. *I'm willing to do my best.*"

Rose laughed. "Great, Gary. That's all it takes."

After our lunch break I wheeled myself back into the healing hut to find Rose sitting quietly in her chair, hands in her lap, staring right through me. I stopped short, at first uncomfortable, then realized she had the same distant look on her face the villagers had when they sat on the ground, staring into space.

Rose took a deep breath and blinked, then smiled at me. "That's right," she replied as if in response to my thoughts. "Aboriginal people spend a lot of time in a meditative state—what's sometimes called Dreamtime." She looked very peaceful. "It's a natural state for us, and it's also one of the tools for controlling what we are focused on, and subconsciously attracting, as I mentioned. Have you ever meditated, Gary?"

"Not that I know of," I joked. "Maybe I'm not 'natural.'"

She grinned. "For us, Dreamtime is vital, part of our way of life."

"I have noticed how often the villagers will sit or stand just staring off into space." I realized with embarrassment that at first I'd thought this meant they weren't very bright. "Is that what you call meditating?"

"Yes, that's it exactly," Rose affirmed. "Meditation doesn't involve finding some special kind of pose and closing your eyes, or even being alone. Meditation is just learning how to relax, go inside, and listen. If you have a problem or a question, just get quiet, go within, and ask and your inner knowing will provide you with an answer. Try it now for a while."

I closed my eyes because that felt more comfortable and private, and tried to reach some kind of peaceful, meditative stance. Instead, I became excruciatingly aware of every distraction—the heat, the sweat trickling down my neck, a kind of dull cramp in my right buttock, the heavy feeling of my hands in my lap. I couldn't ignore the high-pitched sound of children shouting and playing in the village, as if today they were making a special effort to divert my attention. After what seemed an eternity, I opened my eyes a bit to see Rose watching me.

"How was that?" she asked.

"Do you want the truth? I didn't feel a thing. I was aware of every distraction. I guess I'm not meant to be a meditator."

"Don't worry," Rose reassured. "It takes time to learn how to get quiet enough and relaxed enough to really listen. Just stick with it for a while, and you'll be surprised at the results. Meditation is a state of mind, nothing more. The longer you do it, the easier it becomes, and the easier it is for you to avoid negative energy and achieve greater equilibrium."

I wheeled myself outside for a break, and ironically the village was back to its usual quiet condition, no kids running around noisily. I was getting used to these little lessons of life in the Outback by now, so I just "rolled with the flow" and parked myself in the sparse shade of the one scraggly small tree near my hut.

Two women passed by me, carrying some fruit on big leaves. They sat on the ground near the grizzled old man I'd noticed several times watching me at the evening gatherings. As if to demonstrate Rose's lesson of the day, the three of them sat motionlessly gazing past the huts—or perhaps through them toward the openness of the bare landscape. I tried to imagine myself able to feel such a level of peacefulness as they displayed.

A nudge on my arm claimed my attention. It was a young boy whose name I didn't know. Shyly he held out a tablet of the graph paper Ray had brought from town for the children, along with pens for drawing. On the top page was an elaborate geometric design of interconnected lines, stars, and circles, somewhat like the body painting the villagers did for celebrations. The beautiful creation caught me off guard, and I wished I had words in their language to tell him how good it was.

I looked up and the boy was grinning now.

I nodded, "Very good." I started to hand back the tablet.

He pushed it back at me, handing me his pen, indicating with motions that I should add to the drawing.

I didn't want to ruin it, so I shook my head, not knowing if he would understand.

But he insisted, so I took the pen and made some new lines connecting a few of the star designs in a polyhedron. I handed the tablet back to him, and his grin widened. Clutching the tablet to his chest, he ran off to join the little huddle of kids watching from a distance, giggling.

"Good work, Mate." It was Ray. I hadn't heard him come up behind me.

"What was that about?" I tilted my head toward the kids.

Ray just smiled and wheeled me back to the healing hut. "Here he is, Rose. I think he's ready to take another shot at connecting."

Rose and I practiced meditating again for a while. Though I didn't think I was "getting it," I did notice that I wasn't paying as much attention to the stuffy heat inside the hut or the distracting noise of a bird or the kids running past outside.

"Good. Just make it a regular practice, and you'll see. Now let's try something else."

Rose gave me another exercise for creating conscious focus. This was to look at seven areas of my life on a regular basis. She called these the Seven Basic Issues of the Heart.

"All of the problems of the world are variables of these seven. They are: emotional problems, health problems, problems with relationships, finances, sexuality, learning, and spirituality."

"These are the root of all our other problems?" This was too simple an explanation for the kind of turmoil and mess I felt in my life.

Undeterred, Rose continued. "Each one of these issues can cause problems in the other areas. For example, if someone in your culture has a health problem, it might cause you to have financial problems because you have to pay the doctor and relationship problems because you don't feel well enough to relate emotionally to your family and friends. If you have a relationship problem, it might cause you to have financial problems because you can't concentrate on your job or health problems due to the stress.

"When we work on your reprogramming, we will also be working on these seven areas again and again, so just remember them for now and think about them. Try to make positive statements about each area, using *yet* and avoiding *wishing* and *wanting*. Remember, the subconscious mind doesn't know the difference between something real and something envisioned."

That night, as I lay on my plank bed, I thought about Rose's words. I could see that Focus was a tricky one. It was not just a matter of putting my attention on something, it meant being very conscious about what I was putting my attention on. And, more importantly, it was about choosing what I was focusing on.

I had tried to block my mind from focusing on an abusive childhood by numbing myself, keeping myself from feeling. That hadn't worked, because underneath the numbness was always the pain it was attempting to cover. My thoughts turned to my brother Joe, who had also suffered at the hands of my father. Towering at 6' 8" and weighing over 280 pounds, Joe had grown up to be a big man, while my father was only 5' 4" and weighed about 125 pounds. Joe could have put a physical stop to our father's tirades and beatings by the time he was fourteen, but he never found the courage. My father had always been able to intimidate my brother.

And then, in the middle of June on a sunny day in Chicago, Joe found a way to end my father's abuse. My mother was out of town on business, and my wife Tina and I had gone to her house to get some items I had stored in her garage. Joe and his wife were living with my mother at the time, and they had given me a key.

I walked down the pathway between the house and the alley, and my wife followed a few steps behind. As I went to insert the key into the side garage door, it swung open. *That's odd,* I thought. My eyes had not adjusted from the sunlight, but I could see that my mother's car was parked face in. That wasn't right. She always backed her car into the garage.

I felt that something was wrong and told Tina to stay behind. As I stepped into the darkness of the garage, I saw a figure in the car, slumped across the steering wheel. My heart began to beat wildly. It was Joe, his silhouette recognizable even in dim light, with his large frame and his hair cut into a flat top.

I yanked open the door and called his name. "Joe, Joe," I urged. "Wake up!" I slapped him on the chest a couple times, hoping to get a reaction. He didn't move. I tried again. "Joe, get up! Get up! Stop playing around." His body was stiff and unresponsive.

As my eyes adjusted to the dark, I could see Joe's face. His skin had turned to blackened leather. I bolted out of the side door where my wife still stood and fell to my knees on the grass, sobbing.

"What happened?" she asked in a panic.

All I could say was, "It's Joe . . . he's dead."

The loss seemed overwhelming to me, because Joe was the only member of my family I had really loved and been close to. My wife stood by and watched me cry. She had no idea that for the first time in my life, I was crying for myself.

The coroner told us that Joe had been dead for three days when

I finally discovered him. A neighbor reported that he had heard a car running in the garage a couple of days before, but thought nothing of it.

My younger brother and his wife reacted in disbelief to the news. Along with my mother, they refused to believe that Joe had intentionally killed himself, and they fought with the coroner's office to keep the death from being labeled a suicide. They said that Joe often came over to start up Mom's car when she was gone, and he must have fallen asleep by accident and been overcome by the carbon monoxide fumes.

I knew they were only denying, rationalizing, and avoiding the truth. Under pressure, the coroner changed the death certificate to read, "Accidental Death." I knew better. His death was part of our family legacy—a legacy I thought I had avoided until I came face-to-face with multiple sclerosis.

Joe just couldn't keep the voices in his head at bay any longer. He was unable to change what his mind was focusing on. Finally, he chose to silence the voices in the only way he knew how. As I thought about my brother and this last Essential of Healing, I could see the importance of it.

I realized that I had to consciously choose what I wanted to put my attention on. A choice *not* to think about something just didn't work for me. The only way to do this was to numb myself, and that had had terrible repercussions in my life.

My brother's solution was even worse, for he chose to end his life rather than continue facing his painful thoughts. And now I had been given another option—to train my mind to go in another direction, to think about the good—and by doing this, to attract good to me.

It would not be easy to change the habits of a lifetime. But I was determined to do it. My life depended on it. And as I lay there in the stillness of the Outback night, I knew that I had help. I could hear Rose's words in my mind: *All the intelligence in the entire universe is within you, Gary. You just don't know how to access it yet.* That thought gave me hope as I drifted off to sleep.

8

OPERATING MANUAL

The next morning, Rose told me we were ready to begin the deeper and more specific work of healing. The groundwork had been done.

"We had to lay a foundation for the work we're going to begin today," she announced. "First, you needed to understand the basic principle that underlies all Aboriginal healing—that of connectedness. It's the mortar in the foundation that holds everything together. You needed to understand that everything is connected, that what you think impacts how you feel, which impacts how your body reacts."

I nodded. Although this had seemed like a pretty strange concept at first, I was beginning to see that it was true. More important, I was feeling that truth. I thought of the drawing the boy had shared with me and smiled.

Rose smiled, too, and nodded. "You needed to spend some time working with the Five Essentials of Healing," she continued. "These are the bricks of the foundation. And you have seen that they, too, are interconnected. If you're not Willing, you won't be Aware; and you can't Accept what you're not aware of. If you don't Accept it, you can't take Responsibility for it. If you can't take Responsibility, you can't choose to Focus on the good that you want to attract."

I nodded. "So we have the groundwork. Is it time to build a building?"

"It's time. We're actually going to build a belief system that will support health. In the process, we're going to tear down and discard the one that currently is supporting your disease. To use a metaphor from your own culture, we are going to reprogram you."

"So you're saying that I currently am programmed to have this disease?"

"Yes, at some level, you are. You can call it your program, or the script you created for the drama of your life, or your operating manual. Basically, it's what runs you."

I knew that in many ways I was a mystery to myself. "Okay, so let's read the operating manual."

Rose laughed. "We need to start with some background about the nature of reality. First—and this may be hard for your physicist mind to comprehend—all reality is subjective."

I shrugged. "Okay. My physicist mind is open."

"Let me give you an example," she continued. "When most of us smell a rose, we find its aroma pleasing. But imagine if you were made to smell a rose prior to being beaten as a child. Then the smell of a rose would elicit fear and unhappy feelings. So, is a rose innately pleasing or repulsive?"

"I guess it could be either."

"Right. It is only your power of perception that makes it one or the other. So it is with life, Gary. We are not a mechanical body that thinks. We are the thought and intelligence that creates this mechanical body."

"So you are saying that I can use my mind to change what is wrong with my physical body?"

"Yes," Rose stated firmly. "And that is what we plan to do with you. We are going to take the faulty belief system from your mind and replace it with one that will help you to get well. In order to understand why this works, you need to know that our mind is not confined to our brain. It is not even confined to our physical being. Our mind is our energy, our soul, and our universal presence in what a physicist like yourself might term the unified or nonlocal field."

"Because of this, every time we experience an emotion, we not only affect every part of our body, we also affect everyone around us—the entire planet, the entire universe. Every time we think positively, we are healed because we create more healing chemical reactions in our body. Every time we think in the negative, we destroy the body."

"So if I change my thoughts, I can change my body?"

"Yes, but the change has to be on a deep level. It's easy to change on the surface. That's why people go into remission from diseases such as cancer, only to become ill again a few months or years later. For a change to be permanent, it must occur on the cellular level, because the memory of our every experience is locked into that cellular memory."

"Does that imply that our cells have consciousness?" I asked.

Rose looked pleased. "Yes, that's it exactly. It's as if every cell has a little 'brain' of its own that can register emotions. In fact, everything in the universe is alive and conscious. We're surrounded by intelligence, within our body as well as in the outside world. And that intelligence makes up the raw materials from which creation and change can take place."

I let this sink in. It was a very different concept from what I'd always been taught. The brain does the thinking and remembering. The lungs bring in and expel air. The heart pumps blood. The tiny little cells do their tiny little jobs. One big happy team. But consciousness at a cellular level? Cells with feelings and memories?

"Remember how we said that human beings are made up of mind, body, emotions, and spirit?" Rose continued. "This means that when we talk about healing, we mean healing *all* of these parts of us, not just the physical. As I've indicated before, when you squeeze an orange, you get orange juice. What comes out of a human being is the same—you only get what's already in there."

Rose suggested the orange analogy helps to explain why muscle testing works.

"We have seen that the body doesn't lie," she clarified. "It knows our most deeply held beliefs and plays them out in our behavior. And it remembers. Everything that has happened to you in the womb, at birth, and throughout your lifetime is remembered within your body as well as in your mind. Your experiences do not disappear into thin air, but remain locked into the intelligence of your being. These memories held in your body are the basis for your programming."

Although this was a lot to comprehend, I had been impressed by my body's responses during muscle testing. When I tried to tell a lie, like saying my name was something other than Gary, I was unable to hold my arm up. Rose explained that this programming comes not only from our experiences but also from our genetics. In our genes we carry the physical history of our ancestors. So the minute we're conceived we are actually taking on not only the programs of our parents, but those of our grandparents and our great-grandparents, and so on back through time, forever. Our programming continues to develop while our mother carries us in her womb and during birth itself.

"We also receive an emotional inheritance," Rose told me. "Any mother who has more than one child can tell you that each baby comes into this world with a distinct temperament. We do not enter this life as blank slates. Psychologists tell us that by the age of seven, we have already cemented our personality and behavioral patterns, and we run with that program for the rest of our lives. Yet most of us have no conscious awareness of our life before the age of five, the most influential years in our development."

"So how do we discover what the program is, if we don't remember it consciously?" I asked.

"The information is not lost to us," she revealed. "There are techniques by which we can discover how the events of our childhood have affected our present life. We can't undo the experiences of our childhood, but we can reprogram the effects they have on us. We can take an undesirable experience and transform it into a positive result."

At this point I was having difficulty seeing how I could transform my experience of my father or my failed marriages or my alienated children or my MS.

Rose saw this in my eyes. "The effect things have upon us, whether positive or negative, is a matter of choice—how we choose to perceive the situation. It is possible to change one's internal programming in the cells where it resides. In fact, that's what we're going to start today."

"But first we're going to explore your current programming. We're going to read your operating manual. And then we're going to write you a new one."

"Okay. Where do we start?"

"Just where you'd rather not go," Rose answered. "With your emotions."

I groaned.

She laughed. "This is especially important for you, Gary, but you are not alone. Emotions are complex and puzzling for most of us. Society often tells us to be kind and loving, but when our survival is at stake, fear and anger are appropriate. These feelings can help us to survive. But poor programming will cause us to feel anger or fear in situations when it is neither useful nor appropriate."

Rose explained that we would use muscle testing to read my body's current operating manual.

"Your subconscious mind, through your body, will give us the answers we need," she asserted. "I'm going to give you a series of statements that you are to repeat, with your arm extended, just as we did before. It will take time to uncover all the various aspects of your programming, so we will continue working on it for several sessions. Now, let's find out what your body has to tell us."

She paused. "Remember, every time I say 'hold,' breathe out a little bit. Then you won't be using brute strength against me when I try to push down your arm. Repeat after me: *I am willing for good things to happen in my life.*"

I repeated this phrase and Rose easily pushed down my arm.

"See, you are losing energy there. Your body does not believe this. Now say: *I release all guilt and have peace of mind.* And hold. Look at that, your arm is falling again. Say: *I am full of guilt.* See how strong your arm is holding up?"

She was right. I couldn't believe it. Even though my intention was to hold my arm up firmly as she spoke all of these positive statements, it kept wilting like a wet noodle.

"All right, repeat these statements after me:

"I am safe and secure.

"I trust myself and others.

"I am deserving and worthy of only good things in my life.

"I have faith in myself and others.

"I accept myself and others.

"I love myself and others, unconditionally."

My arm collapsed during all of these statements, even when I began trying a little to hold it up, contrary to Rose's instructions.

"Gary, you do not believe any of these statements. Do you know why? It's because you made decisions about yourself early on in your life that determine your present reality. But you must understand that these things are not carved in stone, they are choices. When something happens to us as small children, we make a determination about what that event means to us. For example, you decided that you weren't safe, and that decision has colored everything about your life, making you live fearfully. Now, that belief may have been appropriate from a child's standpoint, especially if you came from a violent household. You may have had good reason to fear for your life. But as an adult, it only keeps you blocked from your true potential, and that block causes you pain. You are stuck viewing life through a child's fearful eyes."

I let her words sink in. I kept remembering the boy sharing his drawing so openly, the other village children laughing and playing in absolute surety of being loved as a vital part of the whole village. I wanted a chance to start over with that faith in life "programmed" in my cells.

Rose was watching me, compassion softening the weathered lines of her face. I met her gaze, and for a moment I could see a light glowing about her, the way I'd seen the villagers the night of my arrival celebration.

She nodded, and then said gently, "Gary, say: *I want to live.*"

"I want to live," I repeated. I really did want another chance. But to my chagrin, my arm collapsed again.

I shook my head in frustration. "All right. To some extent I can see why I don't really believe those other statements," I conceded. "But this last one—I *do* want to live. Why else would I have gone through every-thing I did to get here? Years ago I had a knee injury from football and when I went into surgery, I prayed I wouldn't wake up. At that time in my life I really did want to die. But now I really do want to live," I insisted.

"That's good," she agreed, "but let's see what you really want sub-consciously, say: *I want to die.*"

"I want to die," I repeated. My arm held strong. "Now where did that come from?" I asked, distressed.

"Probably from the time you were conceived," Rose proposed kindly.

She took a deep breath. "Okay, this next statement that I want you to say is rather long: *I respect, appreciate, approve of, nurture, acknowl-edge, praise, support, and thank myself.* And hold."

When my arm fell, Rose concurred, "You don't do any of those things. Now say: *I release all sabotage. I have high self-esteem and a good image.*"

Again my arm fell. "You don't believe those statements, either. Say: *I release all shame and humiliation. I am an emotionally well-adjusted person.*"

My arm collapsed on both of those statements.

"Now say: *I don't have a fear of failure or success.* And hold. Your arm crumbled. You don't believe that one, either."

"It's so strange," I observed. "It's like there's nothing there. I try, but I can't hold my arm up."

Rose nodded. "On a conscious level, you want the positive state-ments to be true. However, your current programming knows they are *not* true. Remember, we are discovering what your *body* believes to be true, the belief system that is lodged in your very cells. That informa-tion comes from a subconscious level.

"Now, let's find out what you believe about your MS. I want you to say *I allow myself to accept and love my MS.* And hold."

As I stated the words, my arm collapsed.

"Now that's what you need to learn to do," suggested Rose.

"I need to learn to *love* my illness?" I questioned.

"Yes," she answered firmly. "You need to love it and accept it, and then it will go away."

It seemed a very tall order. I should love this disease that had crippled me, numbed me, threatened me with death? I didn't think I could. But I affirmed to myself, "I'm willing. That's all I can do right now. But I'm willing."

As always, the day's lessons were on my mind that night as I lay on my hard board bed, looking out at the stars in the blackness of the Outback sky. At the start of the day, I had been very curious to see what was in my operating manual, the script that I had written for my life. It had indeed been enlightening. It had also been horrifying. I was run by shame and guilt. I had no faith in myself. I didn't approve of or appreciate myself. I had a fear of both success and failure. And I didn't want to live.

The only bright spot in this scenario was that a new program could be written, a new owner's operating manual created. As I drifted between wakefulness and sleep that night, I could see it in my mind's eye. The old manual, torn and dirty, in the trash can. A new one, freshly printed, nicely bound, in my hands. I could read the title: *Operating Manual for Gary Holz*. And then the subtitle: *Revised Edition, New and Improved*.

I smiled and went to sleep.

9

A NEW PROGRAM

The next morning I woke to a nice surprise—it was raining. After so many days of dry, dusty heat, it felt like all the parched cells of my body were opening to this gift of moisture. I sat outside my hut, raising my face to the steady rainfall.

The villagers were bustling around, again mostly in silence, positioning tarps to catch the runoff in storage cisterns to use for wash water and cooking. Most of them had taken off their minimal clothing to enjoy the added benefit of a free shower.

"Morning, Mate." Ray ambled over, shirtless, rubbing the stump of his arm as the drops beaded in his wiry hair and slicked over his face. "Beautiful day."

I nodded and held up a palm to cup the raindrops, thinking here was another thing to be grateful for. I was waiting for one of Ray's pithy commentaries on life lessons.

You got it already, Gary. I heard this response clearly in my mind, though Ray hadn't opened his mouth. I looked up at him, startled.

He just grinned and nodded, then stepped around behind me to push me down the path to Rose's healing hut.

For the next several days I worked with Rose to uncover my current belief system, my current programming. One morning she came with a stack of papers in her hand and announced it was time to begin the process of reprogramming.

"We have a lot of material to cover, but I'm not going to ask you to repeat all of it. It would take too long. Since you are a Western person and come from a culture that believes in the written word, I've created several pages of statements designed to test your belief system.

"If you were one of the people in the village, I would work with you telepathically—"

"Telepathically!" I sat staring at her. So it wasn't just my imagination, I really had "heard" that silent response from Ray.

That's right, Gary.

And now I was hearing Rose's "voice" in my head. I concentrated, trying to get a fix on it, but it dissolved into static. I glanced over at Ray, who'd been sitting in on this lesson. He was resting against the wall with his eyes closed, seemingly off in his own world.

Rose smiled. "You're starting to get it, Gary. A lot of our communications here in the village don't require us to speak aloud. You're not quite there yet, but you soon will be. For now, we'll keep working verbally."

She held out a stack of paper with writing on it. "I want you to just glance down these pages. You don't even have to read them. Just fix your eyes on them, and your mind receives the whole lot, as if you were taking a picture of it. I call this the ultimate speed-reading. Now glance at them and hold your arm up."

As she pressed on my arm, it once more collapsed. "You don't believe in any of this," she observed. "You're still fighting me."

"I don't mean to fight you." I was still reeling from the revelation that I could learn to communicate telepathically. And I was trying so hard to think positively that beads of sweat were rolling down my face.

"The next group of statements has to do with your MS." Rose wasn't giving me any slack today. "If we stop and test each one, it's going to take too long, so I'm just going to read these statements to you. And then we'll test some at the end when we're finished. This is the program we're going to put into you. Sometimes I may repeat things a little bit, because I want to make sure I have covered everything."

She started down the list:

"I allow myself to be open to all communication between myself and others.

"I allow myself to communicate with love, joy, peace, and freedom.

"I allow, accept, and love my MS.

"I allow my soul to give myself permission to release the need to have MS."

She tilted her head, studying me, then continued, "Let's test this next one. Repeat after me: *I release all issues . . . regarding mental hardness . . . hard-heartedness . . . inappropriate iron will . . . inflexibility . . . and fear regarding MS."*

I earnestly repeated these phrases after Rose, but when she pushed down on my arm, it still collapsed.

"Oh, shit!" It burst out explosively. "Why can't I get this? I'm trying so hard."

Ray suddenly sat up and opened his eyes, smiling over at me encouragingly. "It's all about choices, Mate," he advised. "You're choosin' to be this way."

"I'll put it another way," Rose added. "We give ourselves permission to feel a certain way, and to hold certain beliefs. No one forces us to act, think, or feel in a certain way. Therefore, you really can *choose* to have loving, joyous thoughts, to make choices with ease and freedom."

"But how?" I pleaded.

"That's what we're working on. That's where your programming comes in. Now, listen to these statements:

"I allow myself to create a loving, joyous, free, and easy life and world.

"I allow myself to feel safe and free to release the MS.

"I allow myself to release all issues in relation to my nervous system and communication process in my life and in my body.

"I allow myself to be open and receptive to all communication from myself and others."

She paused. "Let's test those statements. And hold."

This time, my arm held a little more firmly before sinking down.

"Good, Gary, your strength is getting better. Now, because your nerves have to do with communication, I want you to listen to several programming statements that have to do with communication."

She repeated a long series of affirmations, ending with more statements:

"*I release the need for my immune system to destroy and attack my nervous system and create MS.*

"*I allow myself to open my heart and create only loving communication with myself, others, and my body.*"

Again, my arm felt stronger.

"What did you mean when you said that my nerves had something to do with the way I communicate?" I asked.

"All autoimmune diseases have to do with faulty communication," Rose stated. "MS, especially, because it causes your immune system to attack your nervous system, the lines in your body that carry communication between your brain, your organs, and your cells. It's as if your adult self is abusing your child self for its inadequacies. We need to reshape your programming so that you don't inflict this type of abuse upon yourself. Listen to these statements:

"*I release the need to believe in cruel, selfish, and uncaring behavior toward myself and others.*

"*I release all suppressed aggression and resentment toward my family, father, mother, and others in my life.*

"*I release the need to be immature and childlike by relying upon others to take care of me.*

"Let's test that last statement. Say, *I am immature and avoid my responsibilities.* And hold."

"*I am immature and avoid my responsibilities,*" I declared. My arm held firm, and a feeling of sadness rose up inside of me.

"That's a very strong response," Rose observed, noticing my distress. "Because of your upbringing by your father—because he didn't teach you to be responsible, because he behaved irresponsibly—you took that program from him. That's your deep-seated programming. Now, on a conscious level, you are an intelligent human being who wants to be responsible. However, on a deeper level, you refuse."

"Really?" I was fascinated in spite of myself.

"It's like a battle. Your mind knows you are a responsible human being who needs to do responsible things, but this little kid inside is saying, 'I don't want to be responsible for taking care of me or my life.'

"Now, repeat after me: *I release all suppressed anger and fear regarding not being prepared for the demands of living in an adult world.* And hold.

"See how weak your response was? You aren't prepared to live in an adult world, so there's this resentment inside of you. It's saying, 'I don't want to be a grown-up!' All of these issues have helped create your MS."

"I hear what you're saying," I managed, "but it's hard to believe."

"Yes, I know it is," Rose agreed. "But now that you're aware of these feelings, you're ready to start your healing. We're going to reprogram you so that your inner self is *fully* capable of living and taking responsibility as an adult in an adult world."

She gave me an encouraging look. "Okay, let's try this one. Repeat after me: *I release the need to warehouse anger, resentment, and fear regarding growing and having to be responsible for myself and others. This includes handling all the demands as an adult and giving up dependency upon others.*"

My response to this statement was stronger, and I began to feel a little better.

"Gary, do you know the difference between being independent and interdependent?" Rose asked. "The ultimate position we all want to occupy is to be interdependent. As youngsters, we learn to be independent. As we go through life, we tell ourselves that we should continue this behavior.

"This belief is what causes the little kid inside us to rebel. He wants to do things for himself all the time. If someone wants to help him, he replies, 'I can do that by myself.' The truth is, we need to be able to accept nurturing, support, and caring from others as well. That's being interdependent at the same time as maintaining the ability to be independent."

What she said made sense. All my life, without realizing it, I had struggled to be emotionally independent from others. Relying on another person just wasn't safe. My family and upbringing had taught me that. Better to be able to stand on my own two feet. All of a sudden it hit me—this was the reason why not one of my friends or family members, not even my former wife, had been willing to accompany me to Australia. I had spent a lot of time feeling sorry for myself about it, but the truth was, there wasn't anyone in my life that close to me. I hadn't let them get that close.

Rose spoke, and pulled me from my reverie, "Okay, Gary, repeat these statements after me:

"*I allow myself to complete the dependency cycle I began to learn as a child.*

"*I allow myself to accept adulthood with love, ease, freedom, and joy.*

"*I allow myself to feel safe, secure, responsible, interdependent, and independent both as a child and as an adult.*

"*I allow myself to unlock, accept, resolve, and release all unresolved issues, feelings of dependency, and inadequacy.*

"*I allow the adult within myself to love, accept, and embrace the child within.*" She clarified, "This is to prevent you from continually fighting that little child within yourself in a never-ending, destructive, negative battle."

She continued the list:

"*I release the need to have any neurological difficulties and deficiencies.*

"*I release the need to feel needy and abandoned as a child and now as an adult.*

"*I release all fear of the future and how I will take care of myself.*

"*I allow myself to remove all limitations and boundaries, whether self-imposed or imposed on me as a child by my parents, family, or others.*"

Although I couldn't hold my arm out for all of these statements, it felt stronger on some. That cheered me up a little.

"Now try this one," Rose suggested, relentless: "*I release the need to remove the myelin sheath from my nervous system.*"

My arm wavered. "Is that how I created my MS?" I asked.

"Yes," she replied.

"And it's the myelin sheath that I want to put back on now, right?"

"That's right. Repeat after me: *I allow myself to regenerate the myelin sheath on my nerve fibers. I release the need to paralyze myself.*"

"Is that really possible?" The physicist within me was rising up for one last gasp. "All I have to do is to say it, and it will happen?"

"You can't change your programming through merely repeating positive affirmations," Rose explained. "You must really believe, with your whole soul, the messages behind the affirmations, and live those messages in your daily life, for the reprogramming to be legitimate."

As we ended the session, Rose summed up the heart of the day's lesson: "It's good news and bad news. The bad news is the body remembers and will hold something as true, even when the conscious mind does not. The good news is that you can create new memories for the body, new truths."

Much of the work that remained for me to do in the Outback rested on this concept—that my thoughts and feelings impacted my body on a cellular level, and that it was up to me to consciously and methodically weed out those that did not support my health. In other words, I had to take responsibility for "reprogramming" myself.

Although this was a hard lesson, it was one that gave me hope. If my thoughts could create illness, new thoughts could create health. I was determined to make that happen.

10

SPIRIT GUIDES

I woke up the next morning to chaos. Outside my hut, people were shouting and running past. There was a loud crash, like stacked wood falling. An urgent cry. More pounding feet, as I struggled into my wheelchair and rolled over to the doorway.

People were milling around, pointing, shouting out in a confused babble that sounded all the more startling after the usual calm quiet of the village. Three men holding sharp spears ran past my doorway. I pushed myself outside, craning around to see red dust swirling as some kind of animal dashed around the hunters and barreled back my way. Women and children shrieked and jumped aside, hiding behind huts.

"Back inside, Mate!" It was Ray, running over to push me back into my hut.

I couldn't help leaning past him to see the source of the excitement. It was a wild pig of some kind, dark and bristly, with long, nasty-looking curved tusks. Once I saw those, I let Ray push me back inside.

He was panting. "It's a wild boar; you don't want to mess with him, Gary."

I couldn't help a dig. "So there *was* a dangerous wild animal out there, after all? Not just a kookaburra?"

Very funny. I could hear his voice in my head again.

He shook his head. "The world's still out there, Mate. This doesn't happen too often, but look at it this way, once the hunters catch him, we'll have a feast."

Sure beats more grubs, I thought.

Ray grinned. *We're working on you, Mate.*

In the following days, Rose kept up the work on my "programming." We uncovered the sabotaging beliefs I was holding at a subconscious level and replaced them with ones that would support health and vitality.

The rest of the time, I practiced what I was learning. I noticed more and more the connectedness of everything. I became more willing, more aware, and more accepting. I took responsibility for all that I had created in my life. And I focused on the good that I wanted, in order to set in motion the law of attraction. As a daily practice, I repeated the statements that I wanted to include in my new and revised operating manual.

Although my responses during muscle testing were stronger, I did not see that my MS had changed in any way. Despite this, I felt truly blessed, because I was finding a peace within me that I had never known. I was taking time to sit quietly with the villagers, gazing at nothing more than a rock or a dry bush. Practicing this meditation, I began to feel a part of the Dreamtime shared by the Aboriginal people, began to feel I was connected in the web like that drawing the boy had shared with me.

I was learning patience and was willing for my healing to happen on God's schedule. And I had a growing feeling that there were forces beyond what could be seen and measured with my logical mind, forces that were actively at work in helping me heal. I realized that this feeling had actually started during that evening celebration after I first arrived, when I heard the haunting sound of a didgeridoo.

I had never seen a didgeridoo until I was in Australia and we stopped by Ray's apartment in Brisbane before leaving on our trip to the Outback. In the apartment I saw something crooked leaning in the corner, about ten feet long and six inches in diameter. It looked as if it had been carved out of the branch of a tree.

"What's that?" I inquired.

"That's a didgeridoo," Ray answered. "It's a kind of musical instrument, the one that makes that deep buzzing noise."

Fascinated, I asked, "Could you play it for me?"

"'Fraid not, Mate. It belongs to someone else, a friend of mine. It was made for him, and I'm waiting to give it to him."

"Are you sure he would mind?" I questioned. I knew I was being a little pushy, but I really wanted to hear it.

"Well, it's not a question of I *won't* play it for you. It's that I *can't* play it for you. You see, when somebody makes a didgeridoo, they put a part of their spirit into it. And that part of their spirit stays with the didgeridoo and with the person it was made for.

"Now, you could buy one of these in a tourist shop, but it wouldn't be the same. The ones you'd buy there would be nicer looking than this one, too, because they'd be all straight, whereas this one is crooked. But the real ones take years to make. Only certain trees are used, and there's a ritual involved. And it's only for one person to use, ever."

I'd been disappointed, but as luck would have it, I'd been privileged to hear a didgeridoo right after my arrival in the Outback. It had been like a preview of where this healing work was taking me—that feeling of peaceful connection I'd felt as the haunting song of the wooden instrument filled the air, and I'd glimpsed glowing auras around the villagers.

That had been my first indication that there were things that could not be seen with the eyes, or heard with the ears, but that were real and true. The second indication was Ray's odd habit of having an ongoing conversation with someone who wasn't there, someone he called his "guide," or looking off to the right or left of me as if he were listening to something.

Finally, one day, I asked him what he was doing.

"I'm listening to your spirit guide. Kind of like your guardian angel."

"I have a guardian angel? You mean like in Sunday school?" I joked.

"Why does that surprise you? In your culture children grow up being told they have guardian angels who watch over them in times of need."

"That's true," I concurred, "but by the time we reach adulthood, we no longer talk to invisible entities, and angels just fade away into the realm of fairy tales."

"Well, it seems to me, Mate, that angels have been making a comeback lately, if I can believe all the bestselling books from the U.S. and the TV programs I've been seeing in Brisbane."

Ray was silent for a moment, as if listening to something. "But I don't think people in your culture really understand what angels are all about," he continued. "You mostly see angels as beings that intercede on your behalf in a physical way, maybe saving you from falling off a cliff or from dying in a car wreck. My people see angels as spiritual guides that help you make wise choices.

"Guides are an important part of everyone's life, especially those who need spiritual and physical healing. Once you connect with your guide, it becomes a part of your entire existence, for the rest of your life. Your guide has been patiently waiting to meet you for forty-three years."

"But why didn't we meet earlier, when I was in serious need of a personal angel?"

"Wouldn't you rather ask your guide those questions?"

"You mean I can do that?" I inquired. "Right now?"

"Anytime you're ready," declared Ray. "What do you want to know?"

I thought for a moment. "What does he look like?"

"It's not a 'he,' Mate, it's a 'she.'"

This surprised me. "Not to sound ungrateful, but why a female guide and not a male?"

"Remember your session with Rose where she explained that all of us have both a male and a female side?" Ray asked. "We all have both characteristics inside of us. It's just that, during conception, some of us take on the *physical* characteristics of the male, while the female aspects appear only in our psyche.

"Oftentimes in your culture, as a boy is growing up, his female side is suppressed, intentionally or unintentionally, and he never develops as a whole person. The same is true for women, when their male side is repressed. When this happens, people become ill. You only got to experience your female side early on in your life, before it was crushed. In one way or another you need to reclaim your female side in order to round you out as a person. I'm not talking about gender; I'm talking about being whole."

"That makes sense to me," I agreed. "So, when can I meet this woman?"

"You already have," Ray informed me. "You've just forgotten. She was right there with you in the hospital delivery room when you were born. Whether you've been aware of her or not, she's always been right next to you. She was with you that night in the jazz bar when you were listening to Carolyn. She was the one who put the idea of coming here into your mind. You eventually took her messages to heart, and the result is everything that's happened to you lately."

We were quiet for a minute, while I digested this information. I was fascinated by what he was telling me. Finally I looked up at Ray and saw that his eyes were twinkling as he smiled at me. "Is she good looking?" I blurted out.

Ray shook his head and laughed. "What am I going to do with you, Mate? Yeah, she's good looking. As a matter of fact, if you ever saw her, you'd never look at another woman."

"What's her name?" I inquired.

"Close your eyes, get quiet, and listen for the first name that you hear," Ray answered.

I did what he asked, and it was as if I heard, inside of my head, the name *Julie*.

I reported this to Ray, and he replied, "That's good. From now on, we will refer to her as Julie."

"So, how do I talk to her?"

"Let's start with basic yes and no. Close your eyes and ask Julie to tell you what a 'yes' means. Pay attention to every part of your body, your earlobes, your lips, your torso. She may touch you or send a breath of cool air onto a part of your body."

I did as he asked, trying to meditate and become aware, but after a few minutes I was frustrated. "Nothing's happening."

"Just take it easy and relax," Ray advised. "She doesn't go by your schedule, but by her own."

I closed my eyes again and, three or four minutes later, I felt a gentle but definite sensation of touch on my right earlobe. Excited, I told Ray what had happened.

"Okay, now ask her what a 'no' means."

I patiently waited for a few minutes until I felt something touch me on my left earlobe.

I told Ray, and he nodded in approval. "For the time being, until you get more deeply in touch with your guide, just concentrate on asking questions that can be answered by a yes or a no. But remember, this is just how *your* guide communicates with you. If you ever teach this to someone else, keep in mind that their guide might communicate differently. Talking to your guide is a very personal thing."

"Will I ever be able to actually hear her voice?"

"Eventually you will," Ray affirmed. "It will sound like a gentle voice inside of your head. But for now, just concentrate on creating a rapport with her. I'll leave you alone for a while so that you can start doing that."

I sat there in the quiet heat of the late afternoon, watching the sun move toward the horizon, noticing the companionable warmth I felt in Julie's presence. I thought how far I'd come from the scientist I'd been, who had refused to believe in anything unless someone could empirically prove it to me. Though the old Gary would have found belief in "Julie" irrational, downright crazy, I was beyond caring what that person thought.

My thoughts wandered to the didgeridoo, and I saw a parallel between the making of a "real" didgeridoo and the growth of a human being. A real didgeridoo is endowed with a part of its creator's spirit, and that spirit stays with the didgeridoo and with the person for whom it was created. That spirit is the source of the richness and haunting loveliness of the sound.

I had the thought that each one of us is endowed with part of our Creator's spirit when our bodies are created for us at birth, and that spirit stays with us throughout our lifetime and helps us learn the lessons we need to learn. Some people call that spirit a higher self, a connection to the Universal Power, a Guide, or whatever. For me, that spirit was called Julie, and I knew that I would never be without her presence.

Since that experience in the Outback, I've had many conversations with my Spirit Guide. She is always with me. I am totally convinced that each of us has that help, that comfort, that guidance, and that all we have to do is get quiet enough to hear it. And when we connect with that part of God that is within each of us, our lives become rich and lovely, just like the hauntingly beautiful sound of the didgeridoo.

11

LOVE AND FORGIVENESS

One morning Rose began our session by saying it was time for me to take a very important journey.

"A journey? You mean leave the village?"

"No, it's a journey in the spiritual realm," she answered. "It's a journey we all must take within this lifetime. It's the journey that takes us from being a child to becoming an adult. And what you need to make this journey are the powers of love and forgiveness."

When she mentioned forgiveness, I knew she was talking about my father. Although I had become increasingly grateful for all aspects of my life, I was still not able to feel gratitude about his abusive treatment. There was certainly no gift in my relationship with him.

"So I should just forgive and forget?" I asked. The thought was bitter. It seemed like letting my father get away with all that he had done.

"No," replied Rose. "Human beings actually are constructed so that they cannot forgive and forget. They can't forget, but they can forgive. The body never forgets anything, but we can learn to forgive how it has affected us. We can't erase a memory. But we can change its effect from negative to positive."

"How can I forgive my father after all that he did to me?" I questioned. "And why should I?"

"Because blaming your father is a barrier to being able to give and receive love from others," she explained. "The bottom line is that the world is what it is. When you realize that your mother was the perfect mother for what you needed to learn during this lifetime; that your father was the perfect father to help you to find your strength; and that your brothers, ex-wives, children, business experiences, schooling, and even your MS, were all exactly as they needed to be, then you will be free. You will be free to really be alive. You'll be free to love and accept people instead of judging them.

"Gary, if you're going to heal, it's vital that you forgive anyone who has ever harmed you. You can't forget it. But you can find the gift in it. And you can forgive it. It's important for you to understand this. This is the logic of the heart, the starting point of truly living, of becoming fully involved in this life."

I sat quietly as I tried to grasp what she was telling me. For someone who had spent a lifetime devoted to the hard logic of numbers and facts, the logic of the heart was a difficult concept. I did not see how I could forgive my father. I certainly could not feel gratitude or see the gift in our relationship.

Finally, I let go of trying to analyze her words and just let them be. Seeing that I could not go any further at the time, Rose quietly changed the subject and we continued with the reprogramming process.

It was Ray who brought up my father again, that evening after dinner. Out of the blue, he turned to me and said, "Your father was a pretty good old fella, wasn't he?"

I was sure Rose thought I would talk more freely with Ray about this subject and had put him up to this conversation. I was having none of it. I instantly thought of a time when my brother Tom was about eight years old and I was ten. We were sitting on the floor playing in the living room, when suddenly my father came thundering into the room, knocked my brother flat on his back, and began hitting him while Tom tried to shield himself. I couldn't remember what Tom had done, or even if my father had a reason. Being drunk and full of rage was all the reason he ever needed.

My first response was relief—relief that it was my brother and not me who was getting the beating. Then, all of a sudden, I heard myself yelling at my father to leave my brother alone. I don't know where that courage came from, but it didn't last long. My father turned on me and I ran from the room in terror.

"No," I said adamantly to Ray. "He was not a 'pretty good fella.' He was a drunk who beat the shit out of me, my mother, and my brothers every chance he got."

"Well, he got you into the world, didn't he?" countered Ray.

"So what if he did?" I returned, raising my voice. "He never loved me, and he made my life a living hell."

Ray sighed and shook his head. "Look, Mate, you blame your dad for everything that ever happened to you. It wasn't his fault that he was a drunk. He wasn't a good father to you, but that was also his gift to you. That's how you got so strong so fast, not only emotionally, but in school, in reaction to your dad who never gave you his approval."

I felt sadness welling up inside of me then. And I felt regret. Regret that my father and I had never been friends, had never been able to talk even once before he died.

"But why did he have to drink himself to death?" I asked. "Why did he have to destroy his life and that of those around him?"

Ray looked at me with compassion. "I know your father was weak, Gary. He was faced with a wall in his life—his alcoholism—and that wall stopped him. Your wall was your diagnosis, your death sentence, but you are trying to get over your wall. I know how tough it was for you to get on that airplane with no support from your family and friends. No one was willing to go with you, and yet you got on that plane anyway. That took a lot of courage.

"Your father didn't have that kind of courage, but there are still things you can be grateful for. You've been carrying your feelings about him in your body for a long time now, and your body is crumbling under the load. So it's time to look at forgiveness. Without forgiveness, it may be impossible to get well. Just think about that tonight before you go to sleep."

That night as I lay on my sleeping board, listening to the now familiar sounds of the Outback, I continued to think about my father—about the alcohol, about the beatings, about the abuse. And I thought about my father's early death. I had still been in the Army when I received notification that he was ill and in the hospital. An emergency leave of absence was set up for me to return home, but I really didn't want to go. Somehow, I already knew what I would find.

My father had never been a large man, but now his illness had reduced him to a shell. Like many alcoholics, he had cirrhosis of the liver. He was only fifty-seven years old, but he looked ancient, skeletal and frail, in the hospital bed. The doctor told him he had to stop drinking or he would be dead in six months.

He didn't stop drinking, and in five months he was gone. We buried him on Christmas Eve.

As those thoughts drifted through my mind, I thought about the kookaburra bird, a small bird with a very scary call. I thought about forgiveness. And something shifted. There was no magical transformation—I didn't instantly let go of all my anger and feel a great love for my father—but after a while, I felt a little lighter, a little more peaceful. And with that, I went to sleep and slept soundly.

The next morning, Rose told me she had prepared a special program that would help remove all of those fears buried within me so that I would be ready to trust all the statements we had worked on for the past few days.

"We're going to program in more positive statements and remove more of the negative programming embedded in the cells of your body," she said. "And we're going to do this in a very interesting way."

"What are you going to do?"

"Did you know that your body can read?" Rose asked. "That's how we're going to do it. We're going to let your body read."

I was mystified.

"Let me show you how this works," Rose explained. "I have two pieces of paper here. I'll put your name 'Gary' on one piece and the name 'Bill' on another, just as we did in the muscle testing. Then I'll put each paper, one at a time, on your chest. Your body knows the difference between what is written on each piece of paper by the energy they carry, the negative and positive energy associated with true and untrue statements. Once more, I need you to lift your arm. It will tell us, by holding strong, which paper contains your name."

Rose slipped one of the pieces of paper on my bare chest under my shirt. "Your arm is weak with this paper." She switched papers and continued, "And strong with this one. Look at this paper. It reads 'Gary.'"

"That's pretty amazing." I was impressed. "Do you do this when you work with other Aboriginal people, or is this just for me?"

"This is just for you, Gary. I would work with my own people telepathically. But this will work for you, believe me. Now that you get the idea, I am going to place these pages on your body, so you will be able to absorb all of this information. The statements written on these pages will help you to eliminate antagonism, anger, resentment, hostility, and similar negative energies. Instead, you'll be programmed for positive beliefs and emotions."

"Can I read what's on the papers?"

"Absolutely not," Rose objected. "In fact, if you do, you will sabotage the entire program. The key to reprogramming is circumventing your conscious mind and speaking directly to your subconscious mind. If you read what is on the papers, your conscious mind will find a way to get around the statements, and you will be right back where you started."

"Okay, I won't look," I promised.

Rose instructed me to lift myself out of my chair and lie down on a plank bed like the one in my hut. I was so nervous about accidentally reading what was on the papers that I squeezed my eyes tightly shut.

"Now, I'm just going to place a towel on your stomach so the pages don't fall off. I want you to relax, focus, and absorb the reprogramming. It'll help if you can go into a meditative state."

Rose slipped a thick stack of papers under my shirt and arranged them in the center of my chest, over my heart. Then she and Ray quietly left the room. I lay there listening to the sounds of the villagers, trying to still my mind. What Rose had said about my body knowing how to read seemed strange to me. I felt the part of myself that was the physicist trying to slip back in and sabotage me. But I couldn't let him. I had come too far.

After what seemed to me like a very long time, Rose returned, took the papers off my chest, and asked me to sit up. "How do you feel?" she inquired.

"Fine, but strange," I muttered, at a loss for words to describe my experience.

She looked at me closely. "Good," she commented. "Now, let's continue with the testing to discover your programming." For the next hour or so, she continued muscle testing, asking me to listen to some statements and to repeat others, as she had the days before. Finally, she seemed satisfied.

"Okay, Gary, that's great. You're doing well, and I'm very pleased with your progress."

After we broke for a light lunch, Rose was ready with another stack of papers to be "read" by my body. But first, she indicated that we needed to talk a bit more about forgiveness.

I thought about my father, and noticed that I didn't have the immediate flash of resentment that I usually did. I didn't feel love, but on the other hand, I didn't feel hatred either. It was strange.

"Gary, do you understand how forgiveness comes in?" Rose continued. "It is the antidote to blame. By forgiving others, the forgiver is the one who is freed. Often, once we have forgiven someone, it's as if a load of bricks has fallen off our back. This is because anger and blame carry such negative energy.

"And just as you must learn how to forgive others, you must also learn how to forgive yourself. Learn to accept that everything, including the pain you feel in your life, is for a greater purpose—to help you discover who you really are and what you are here on this earth to do."

As I listened, I began to realize what it was costing me to carry around my anger at my father. I truly wanted that "load of bricks" off my back. I wanted to free myself.

"I hear what you're saying, Rose. And I don't know if I can do it—forgive others, even forgive myself. I don't know if I can. But I'm willing."

"That's all anyone can ask, Gary," she remarked. "Now, I'm going to put a program on your chest that will help with this. Lie quietly and relax. Think about what you have learned today, and Ray will return in a while to check on you."

I closed my eyes and drifted into quietness and peace. I don't know how much time passed, for I seemed to have slipped into a place that was timeless. Finally, as the afternoon began to wind down, Ray returned. He touched my foot to wake me and, for a moment, I thought I felt the warmth of his hand. Attributing this feeling to my dreamlike state, I let it pass.

"How do you feel?" Ray asked.

"Peaceful," I murmured.

Ray nodded and lowered himself to sit on the dirt floor near me, closing his eyes. We were quiet for a while, but it was a very "full" silence, and I was aware of a strong connection to him.

Something—like a footfall but inside my head—made me open my eyes to see Ray looking up at an empty space between us. At that moment, an old Aboriginal man appeared standing there. He was very dark, with wiry white hair and beard. He was looking at me with the most luminous gaze I had ever seen.

Startled by this sudden apparition that looked very much solid, and *real*, I struggled to sit up.

"Be at peace," the old man told me, only he wasn't moving his lips. I could hear his voice in my mind. He smiled. "I am glad that I have finally met you."

The old man held my gaze for a moment longer, and then he was gone.

I fell back down to lie there stunned. I knew my old reality would label me crazy, but I also knew with absolute certainty that the visitor was real. I felt his presence still within me, calm and solid.

"Congratulations, Mate," Ray confided quietly.

I looked over to see him nodding. "What—who was that?" I asked.

"That's Old Healer. He's been waiting for you to be able to see him."

I took a deep breath. "Does he live in the village? I haven't seen him before."

"He did live here. He was a great healer, Gary. He passed on fifty years ago, but he still visits me in Dreamtime. He's the one who told me you'd be coming here."

I'd learned too much to deny the reality of what he was saying. I felt its truth in my heart.

"Well, here we go, then. Time to get you some dinner." Ray, pragmatic as ever, rose and stepped over to help me. He touched my foot and again I thought I felt the barest contact in my numb extremity.

Ray took me back to my hut in companionable silence, and then went to get my dinner.

Once there, I realized that I needed to take care of my catheter. To do this, I had to go to a small outhouse, located nearby, for some privacy. As I wheeled myself there, I distinctly felt the urge to urinate. This couldn't be a real sensation, I told myself. I had absolutely no bladder control and wore a catheter that went directly into my bladder to drain it as needed. But the excitement of the possibility that I might be feeling a tiny bit of sensation in my body would not leave me. I hurried as fast as I could along the narrow dirt path that led to my destination.

Once I reached the outhouse, I grabbed my cane from the back of the wheelchair and proceeded to drag myself forward using the wall of the building and the cane for support. The few steps inside were slow and cumbersome as I fumbled to keep my balance. Leaning most of my weight against the wall, I began the process of taking care of my catheter.

As I reached out to check the insertion point in my penis, I felt the touch of my hand sear through me with incredible warmth. *It can't be!* I thought. My mind must be tormenting me and playing tricks on me. I braced myself against the wall, allowed my cane to drop, and began to pull out the catheter tube. With every inch, I felt its removal from my body.

As the physical sensation of actually being able to feel something again continued to escalate, the impact of what was happening came flooding into my whole being. I felt filled with love, as if I were catching a glimpse of my life through God's eyes. I experienced clarity of understanding that I had never touched on before.

In a burst of insight I realized that everything I had thought was important—the pursuit of money, success, and material possessions—was meaningless and empty. All my life had been spent in the absence of feeling. I'd been merely going through the motions and missing out on joy, sorrow, love, forgiveness, and compassion—the very cornerstones of life. And now I saw clearly that what really mattered was the simple human ability to feel.

I fell to my knees in the dirt of the outhouse floor. I felt laughter rising inside of me, and I knew what my life and my MS had been trying to teach me—that there is beauty and perfection to be found even in tragedy and pain. I thought I'd been playing the tune of my life alone, but all along I'd been in the middle of a fully orchestrated symphony with a glorious conductor. The keyhole through which I glimpsed my life now became an open door. Everything was possible. I was within the loving arms of my God.

The moment when I began to regain the feeling in my body was the moment that I truly passed over the threshold from death to life. Although I had had powerful experiences working with Ray and Rose, nothing had shaken me to my core—had made me truly consciously believe that I was really going to live—like the feeling of that catheter searing through my penis.

I had come full circle. The numbness in my manhood had been what finally convinced me to go to the doctor many years ago. Now, the first part of me to live again, to feel alive again, was my manhood. I saw that as my past and present were being healed, my entire future was being rewritten. I was not the man I'd been when I'd first gotten off that plane in Brisbane. I was reborn.

With tears of joy on my cheeks, I hollered for Ray.

"What happened?" He came running up to me.

I handed him my catheter and told him that I could feel again. Ray's face lit up with joy. "Gary, you've done it! You're finally getting out of your head. What did I tell you? Was it a long trip?"

"It took a lifetime," I exclaimed, laughing and crying at the same time.

At that moment Ray shouted out what I can only describe as a chant of celebration in his own language. I don't know what he said, but everyone in the village came running. The whole group—men, women, and children—hurried toward us and began whooping with joy. They patted me on the back as they learned the news and, even though I didn't understand the language, I knew they were telling me how happy they were for me.

I'd known that the village was behind me since the night they'd sincerely welcomed me by having a special gathering in my honor, but I'd never expected them to share my happiness so intensely and personally. The way they smiled, patted me on the back, and held my hands, you would have thought that I was their brother, their father, their son. I had never felt such a sense of belonging, and I cried fresh tears.

"What's going on?" Rose asked, hurrying over to us.

Outrageous and earthy as always, Ray replied, "Here, Gary has a souvenir for you," and handed her the catheter. She laughed and shook her head as Ray told her what had happened to me.

"This is wonderful," she beamed. "Oh, Gary, I'm so happy for you."

There was no question of doing any more healing work that day. Instead, we had an impromptu celebration and sat around eating, talking, laughing, and telling stories. I was the man of the hour, and no one seemed to be able to get enough of touching me and sharing in my happiness. That night the people of the village seemed like a living rainbow to me, a rainbow of skin colors from almost white, to brown, to black—indescribably beautiful in their love for me and for one another.

When the young men brought out their bowl of clay body paint and started decorating themselves for the celebration and dancing, one of them turned to me. He tilted his head and smiled into my eyes.

Yes. As I accepted the invitation, his grin broadened.

I pulled off my shirt, and they painted my pale skin with the same lines and dots they wore, a web of connection to life and loving. I was part of the family.

That night, when I lay down to sleep, I experienced a deep sense of well-being. In my days in the Outback, I had come to know the grace of acceptance, but now I was filled with the euphoria of hope. I knew with an unshakable certainty that I was going to get well, and I thanked God.

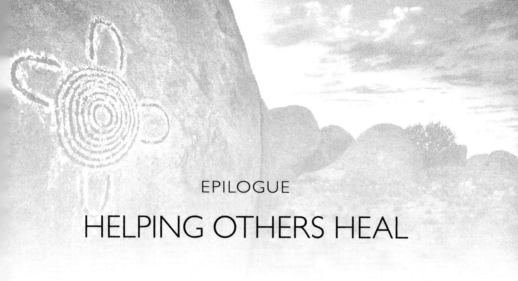

HELPING OTHERS HEAL

When I made my trip to the Outback, I simply wanted to be healed. I didn't know that I would become a healer as well.

After I had completed my studies and healing work with Rose and Ray, the entire village gathered for one more celebration. This was my "graduation ceremony," as I was able to communicate telepathically with all of them by now. Joining in the silent web of connection was one of the most powerful and joyful experiences of my life.

"Gary, you will do well." I heard this gentle voice in my head and looked over to see that Old Healer had joined the circle. Ray seemed to be aware of him there, but it wasn't clear if anyone else saw him.

The grizzled old man nodded and smiled. *"Go out into the world to use your healing gifts. Help others as you have been helped."*

A few weeks after my arrival in the Outback in 1994, I returned to the States on a flight that was dramatically different from the one that had brought me to Australia. Instead of being confined to my wheelchair and my own thoughts, I was able to clumsily walk around the plane, supporting myself on seat backs as I uncharacteristically chatted happily with fellow passengers.

Upon my return I realized that although my life's passion in the past had been as a scientist and inventor, I now had a deep yearning to help others heal as I had been healed. I knew that furthering my education would add to my credibility in bringing these Aboriginal healing techniques to the Western world, so I obtained a Doctorate in Immunology and a Master's Degree in Nutrition.

Since then, I have had the privilege and joy of assisting numerous people in their healing process, including those with AIDS and advanced-stage cancers. They understood not only that their bodies had tremendously powerful healing capabilities but that the healing journey was a process that totally involved mind, body, spirit, and, most importantly, help and assistance from the Big Guy.

My healing process with multiple sclerosis continues. I can tell you that its "challenges" have been the source of some of the best and some of the worst times of my life, but I know they were necessary to bring me to the point where I am now in my life: healing in body and spirit, happily remarried, stronger in my relationships with my grown children, embracing emotions rather than numbing myself to them, and appreciating not only this God-given body but the multiple sclerosis as well.

Although I am most grateful for this healing gift, I know I am merely a conduit for healing. Ultimately, I know that the Big Guy is in charge.

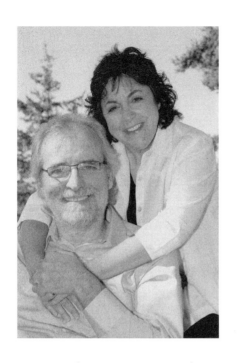

ABOUT THE AUTHORS

Gary Holz, D.Sc., was a physicist, multiple patent holder, founder of high-tech aerospace company Holz Industries, and successful businessman. Dr. Holz authored over 100 articles ranging in topics from alternative medicine to high-energy physics. After his own healing experience with the Aborigines in 1994, he returned from the Outback and became a psychoneuroimmunologist, nutritionist, lecturer, and holistic healer. He resided in the Pacific Northwest with his wife Robbie until his passing in 2007.

Robbie Holz is an international speaker, award-winning author, and holistic wellness consultant living in the Seattle area. She is currently writing the sequel to *Secrets of Aboriginal Healing,* which explores how she and her husband Dr. Gary Holz helped many people successfully restore their health. This forthcoming book also recounts Robbie's own recovery from Hepatitis C, highlights her subsequent experiences with Outback Aborigines, and expands the Aboriginal healing principles into everyday practicality. Visit her website at

www.holzwellness.com.

CONTINUING THE JOURNEY

We invite you to contact us at **info@holzwellness.com**, or you can visit **www.holzwellness.com** to continue your experience through our website, where you can:

- Read about the sequel to *Secrets of Aboriginal Healing*

- Share your insights and read what others are saying

- Learn more about the remote Australian Outback Aborigines

- Communicate with coauthor Robbie Holz

- Integrate the Aboriginal healing steps into your life with Robbie's online course

- Discover more tips on creating a happier, healthier life

- Invite Robbie Holz to speak to your organization

- Read Robbie Holz's blog

- Purchase additional copies of *Secrets of Aboriginal Healing*